# Fibrin Sealing in Surgical and Nonsurgical Fields

Volume **8**

G. Schlag  W. Wayand (Eds.)

# Endoscopy

With 23 Figures, Some in Color
and 16 Tables

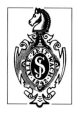

Springer-Verlag
Berlin  Heidelberg  New York
London  Paris  Tokyo
Hong Kong  Barcelona
Budapest

Univ.-Prof. Dr. GÜNTHER SCHLAG

Ludwig-Boltzmann-Institut
für experimentelle und klinische Traumatologie
Donaueschingenstraße 13, 1200 Wien
Austria

Univ.-Prof. Dr. WOLFGANG WAYAND

AKH Linz, II. Chirurgie
Krankenhausstraße 9, 4020 Linz
Austria

ISBN 3-540-58282-7 Springer-Verlag Berlin Heidelberg New York

CIP data applied for

© Springer-Verlag Berlin Heidelberg 1995
Printed in Germany

Production: PRO EDIT GmbH, 69126 Heidelberg, Germany
Typesetting: Mitterweger Werksatz GmbH, 68723 Plankstadt, Germany
SPIN: 10428200        23/3130 5 4 3 2 1 0 – Printed on acid-free paper

# Preface

These eight volumes, which developed out of the international congress "Update and Future Trends in Fibrin Sealing in Surgical and Nonsurgical Fields" held in November 1992, present the state of the art in fibrin sealing. Initially, fibrin sealant played an important role in surgery. During the past few years, it has been increasingly applied nonsurgically and we can now say that it has become an integral component of medical treatment.

The doubts which have been raised by nonusers about the efficacy of fibrin sealant are no longer valid. The correct indication and technique continue to be basic prerequisites for effective treatment. Even today 20 years after fibrin sealant was first used – the three most prominent effects of fibrin sealant are still hemostasis, sealing of the wound, and support of wound healing.

The problems posed by the transmission of viral infections have gained substantially in importance because of the potential transmission of AIDS via fibrin sealant. Fortunately, this is so unlikely today that it no longer represents a cause for concern, which does not mean, however, that research in this field can be discontinued.

Seven years have passed since the last series of books on fibrin sealing were published. Since then many new results have been obtained and clear indications for the use of fibrin glue have developed. Improved optic systems have changed the diagnosis and therapy of gastrointestinal and pulmonary diseases to an extraordinary degree. As in Jules Verne's science fiction novel about the journey to the moon, the reality can catch up with the imagination, and we now have both flexible and rigid intracavitary endoscopes for use in minimally invasive endoscopy, a procedure which has developed from a diagnostic to an operative method. When entering new territory, it is all the more reassuring to have a reliable adjuvent such as fibrin sealant. The table of contents illustrates the large variety of indications.

We, the editors, would like to thank all the authors for their cooperation and excellent contributions and photographs. Their work has made publication of these eight volumes on fibrin sealing possible. Special thanks are due to Dr. V. Gebhardt and his expert colleagues for efficient and constructive cooperation in the publication of these books at the Springer publishing company and to Gudrun Schrodt for her untiring efforts in obtaining manuscripts, proof reading, and corresponding with the authors.

G. SCHLAG
W. WAYAND

# Contents

Endoscopic Fibrin Sealing in Gastroduodenal Ulcer Hemorrhage
G. HEROLD, G. PRECLIK, and E. F. STANGE . . . . . . . . . . . . . . . . . . . . 1

Endoscopic Injection Therapy of Gastroduodenal Ulcer Hemorrhage:
A Randomized Comparison of Fibrin Sealant vs. Polidocanol
R. SALM, K. E. GRUND, J. SONTHEIMER, A. BUSTOS, and E. WEBER . . . . . . 8

Submucosal Fibrin Adhesion in Upper Gastrointestinal Bleeding
J. LABENZ, U. PEITZ, M. WIECZOREK, and G. BÖRSCH . . . . . . . . . . . . . 15

Laparoscopic Surgical Treatment of Duodenal Ulcer Disease
J. MOUIEL, N. KATKHOUDA, and L. IOVINE. . . . . . . . . . . . . . . . . . . . 20

Fibrin Sealing of the Liver Bed After Laparoscopic
Cholecystectomy: A Prospective Randomized Study
P. SCHRENK, R. WOISETSCHLÄGER, and W. WAYAND . . . . . . . . . . . . . . . 30

Endoscopic Application of Fibrin Glue in the Treatment
of Anastomotic Defects, Perforation, and Fistulas in the
Gastrointestinal Tract
H. GROITL, T. HORBACH, R. STANGL, and J. SCHEELE . . . . . . . . . . . . . . 33

Fibrin Sealing in Laparoscopic Colorectal Surgery
T. RECK, C. SCHNEIDER, I. SCHNEIDER, I. GASTINGER,
and F. KÖCKERLING . . . . . . . . . . . . . . . . . . . . . . . . . . . . . . . . . 38

The Use of Fibrin Glue in Sclerotherapy for Esophageal Varices:
Preliminary Results of a Controlled Prospective Study
F. RUCKTÄSCHEL, K. ZIEGLER, and T. ZIMMER. . . . . . . . . . . . . . . . . . 44

Therapy of Gastrointestinal Fistulas with Fibrin Sealant
M. JUNG and B. C. MANEGOLD . . . . . . . . . . . . . . . . . . . . . . . . . . . 50

Endoscopic Approaches for Occlusion of Fistulas
V. LANGE, G. MAIWALD, T. SOUVATZI, and G. MEYER . . . . . . . . . . . . . . 58

Fistulas in Crohn's Disease as a Complication of the Underlying Disease
A. EIMILLER . . . . . . . . . . . . . . . . . . . . . . . . . . . . . . . . . . . . . . 65

Technical Description and Results of Endoscopic Treatment
of Various Solitary Rectal Ulcer Syndrome Pictures
A. EDERLE, G. BULIGHIN, S. PILATI, and S. DESIDERI . . . . . . . . . . . . . .    69

The Occlusion of Anal Fistulas in Crohn's Disease
N. WOLF, I. SCHNEIDER, K. THALER, and C. SCHNEIDER. . . . . . . . . . . . .    75

Human Fibrin Sealants and Postoperative Fistulas: 25 Cases
V. COSTANTINO, A. ALFANO D'ANDREA, and S. PEDRAZZOLI . . . . . . . . . . .    78

Fibrin Sealant in Endoscopic Gynecological Surgery
J. F. H. GAUWERKY . . . . . . . . . . . . . . . . . . . . . . . . . . . . . .    82

Fibrin Sealing in Endoscopic Surgery
D. WALLWIENER, S. RIMBACH, D. POLLMANN, W. STOLZ, J. F. H. GAUWERKY,
and G. BASTERT . . . . . . . . . . . . . . . . . . . . . . . . . . . . . . .    90

Endoscopic Modification of the Marshall-Marchetti-Krantz Operation
D. WALLWIENER, S. RIMBACH, E. M. GRISCHKE, J. JANKY,
and G. BASTERT . . . . . . . . . . . . . . . . . . . . . . . . . . . . . . .    96

Minimally Invasive Lung Surgery: Preliminary Results
W. WAYAND, R. WOISETSCHLÄGER, and R. RIEGER . . . . . . . . . . . . . . .   100

Liver Biopsy: Modified Menghini and Trucut Needles for Fibrin Sealing
of the Biopsy Channel: Clinical Experience
G. JUDMAIER, W. VOGEL, H. P. DINGES, and K. ZATLOUKAL . . . . . . . . . .   106

Subject Index . . . . . . . . . . . . . . . . . . . . . . . . . . . . . . . .   109

# List of Contributors

Alfano D'Andrea, A.
Istituto di Semeiotica Chir. dell'Università
Via Facciolati 71, 35135 Padova, Italy

Bastert, G.
Ruprecht-Karls-Universität, Frauenklinik,
Voßstraße 9, 69115 Heidelberg, Germany

Börsch, G.
Medizinische Klinik, Elisabeth-Krankenhaus,
Akademisches Lehrkrankenhaus, Universität Essen,
Moltkestraße 61, 45138 Essen, Germany

Bulighin, G.
Serv. d. Endoscop. Digest., Osped. d. Villafranca,
37069 Villafranca (Verona), Italy

Costantino, V.
Istituto di Semeiotica Chir. dell'Università,
35135 Padova, Italy

Bustos, A.
Abteilung Allgemeine Chirurgie mit Poliklinik,
Chirurgische Universitätsklinik,
Hugstetter Straße 55, 79106 Freiburg, Germany

Desideri, S.
Serv. d. Endoscop. Digest, Osped. d. Villafranca,
37069 Villafranca (Verona), Italy

Dinges, H. P.
Institut für Pathologie, Universität Graz,
Auenbruggerplatz 25, 8036 Graz, Austria

EDERLE, A.
Serv. d. Endoscop. Digest. Osped., 37069 Villafranca (Verona), Italy

EIMILLER, A.
Sonnenstraße 7, 80331 München, Germany

GASTINGER, I.
Chirurgische Abteilung, Klinikum Suhl, 98527 Suhl, Germany

GAUWERKY, J. F. H.
Ruprecht-Karls-Universität, Frauenklinik,
Voßstraße 9, 69115 Heidelberg, Germany

GRISCHKE, E. M.
Ruprecht-Karls-Universität, Frauenklinik
Voßstraße 9, 69115 Heidelberg, Germany

GROITL, H.
Chirurgische Klinik mit Poliklinik der Universität,
Maximiliansplatz 10, 91054 Erlangen, Germany

GRUND, K. E.
Abt. Allgemeine Chirurgie, Universitätsklinik, Hoppe-Seyler-Straße 3,
72076 Tübingen, Germany

HEROLD, G.
Medizinische Klinik der Universität, Abteilung Innere Medizin I,
Robert-Koch-Straße 8, 89081 Ulm, Germany

HORBACH, T.
Chirurgische Klinik mit Poliklinik der Universität,
Maximiliansplatz 10, 91054 Erlangen, Germany

IOVINE, L.
Univ. de Nice-Sophia Antipolis, Serv. de Chir. Digest.,
Vidéo-Chir. et Transplant.
Hôpital Saint-Roch, 06006 Nice Cedex 1, France

JANKY, J.
Ruprecht-Karls-Universität, Frauenklinik,
Voßstraße 9, 69115 Heidelberg, Germany

JUDMAIER, G.
Abteilung für Intensiv-Medizin, Universität Innsbruck,
Anichstraße 35, 6020 Innsbruck, Austria

JUNG, M.
Johann-Wolfgang-Goethe-Universität, Med. Klinik II,
Abt. Gastroenterologie, Theodor-Stern-Kai 7,
60596 Frankfurt/M., Germany

KATKHOUDA, N.
Univ. de Nice-Sophia Antipolis, Serv. de Chir. Digest,
Vidéo-Chir. et Transplant.
Hôpital Saint-Roch, 06006 Nice Cedex 1, France

KÖCKERLING, F.
Chirurgische Klinik der Universität Erlangen,
Maximiliansplatz 2, 91054 Erlangen, Germany

LABENZ, J.
Medizinische Klinik, Elisabeth-Krankenhaus,
Akademisches Lehrkrankenhaus, Universität Essen,
Moltkestraße 61, 45138 Essen, Germany

LANGE, V.
Schloßpark-Klinik, Chirurgische Abteilung,
Heubnerweg 2, 14059 Berlin, Germany

MAIWALD, G.
Chirurg. Klinik Großhadern, Ludwig-Maximilians-Universität,
Marchioninistraße 15, 81366 München, Germany

MANEGOLD, B. C.
Klinikum der Stadt Mannheim, Fakultät für Klinische Medizin der
Universität Heidelberg, Theodor-Kutzer-Ufer, 68167 Mannheim,
Germany

MEYER, G.
Chirurg. Klinik Großhadern, Ludwig-Maximilians-Universität,
Marchioninistraße 15, 81366 München, Germany

MOUIEL, J.
Univ. de Nice-Sophia Antipolis, Serv. de Chir. Digest.
Vidéo-Chir. et Transplant. Hôpital Saint-Roch,
06006 Nice Cedex 1, France

PEDRAZZOLI, S.
Istituto di Semeiotica Chir. dell'Università,
Via Facciolati 71, 35135 Padova, Italy

PEITZ, U.
Medizinische Klinik, Elisabeth-Krankenhaus,
Akademisches Lehrkrankenhaus,
Universität Essen, Moltkestraße 61,
45138 Essen, Germany

PILATI, S.
Serv. d. Endoscop. Digest., Osped. d. Villafranca,
37069 Villafranca (Verona), Italy

POLLMANN, D.
Ruprecht-Karls-Universität, Frauenklinik,
Voßstraße 9, 69115 Heidelberg, Germany

PRECLIK, G.
Medizinische Klinik der Universität, Abteilung Innere Medizin I,
Robert-Koch-Straße 8, 89081 Ulm, Germany

RIEGER, R.
II. Chirurgische Abteilung, AKH,
Krankenhausstraße 9, 4020 Linz, Austria

RECK, Th.
Chirurgische Klinik der Universität Erlangen,
Maximiliansplatz 2, 91054 Erlangen, Germany

RIMBACH, S.
Ruprecht-Karls-Universität, Frauenklinik,
Voßstraße 9, 69115 Heidelberg, Germany

RUCKTÄSCHEL, F.
Freie Universität Berlin, Universitäts-Klinikum Steglitz,
Abteilung für Innere Medizin und Gastroenterologie,
Hindenburgdamm 30, 12203 Berlin, Germany

SALM, R.
Abt. Allgemeine Chirurgie mit Poliklinik, Universitätsklinik,
Hugstetter Straße 55, 79106 Freiburg, Germany

SCHEELE, J.
Chirurgische Klinik mit Poliklinik der Universität,
Maximiliansplatz 10, 91054 Erlangen, Germany

SCHNEIDER, C.
Chirurgische Klinik der Universität Erlangen,
Maximiliansplatz 2, 91054 Erlangen, Germany

SCHNEIDER, I.
Chirurgische Klinik der Universität Erlangen,
Maximiliansplatz 2, 91054 Erlangen, Germany

SCHRENK, P.
2nd Surg. Unit AKH Linz und Ludwig-Boltzmann-
Institut für Operative Laparoskopie,
Krankenhausstraße 9, 4020 Linz, Austria

SONTHEIMER, J.
Abt. Allgemeine Chirurgie mit Poliklinik, Universitätsklinik,
Hugstetter Straße 55, 79106 Freiburg, Germany

SOUVATZI, T.
Chirurg. Abteilung, Kreiskrankenhaus, Santer-Straße 96,
87616 Marktoberdorf, Germany

STANGE, E. F.
Klinik für Innere Medizin, Medizinische Universität zu Lübeck,
Ratzeburger Allee 160, 23562 Lübeck, Germany

STANGL, R.
Chirurgische Klinik mit Poliklinik der Universität,
Maximiliansplatz 10, 91054 Erlangen, Germany

STOLZ, W.
Ruprecht-Karls-Universität, Frauenklinik,
Voßstraße 9, 69115 Heidelberg, Germany

THALER, K.
Chirurgische Abteilung der Universität Erlangen,
Maximiliansplatz 10, 91054 Erlangen, Germany

VOGEL, W.
Universitätsklinik für Innere Medizin, Anichstraße 35,
6020 Innsbruck, Austria

WALLWIENER, D.
Ruprecht-Karls-Universität, Frauenklinik,
Voßstraße 9, 69115 Heidelberg, Germany

WAYAND, W.
AKH Linz, II. Chirurgie und Ludwig-Boltzmann-Institut
für Operative Laparoskopie, Krankenhausstraße 9,
4020 Linz, Austria

WEBER, E.
ehem. Leiter der Abteilung Biostatik des Deutschen
Krebsforschungszentrums,
69115 Heidelberg, Germany

WIECZOREK, M.
Medizinische Klinik, Elisabeth-Krankenhaus, Akademisches
Lehrkrankenhaus, Universität Essen, Moltkestraße 61, 45138 Essen,
Germany

WOISETSCHLÄGER, R.
AKH Linz, II. Chirurgie und Ludwig-Boltzmann-Institut
für Operative Laparoskopie, Krankenhausstraße 9,
4020 Linz, Austria

WOLF, N.
Krankenhaus Cochem, Abteilung für Chirurgie,
Klosterberg 1, 56812 Cochem, Germany

ZATLOUKAL, K.
Institut für Pathologie, Universität Graz, Auenbruggerplatz 25,
8036 Graz, Austria

ZIEGLER, K.
Freie Universität Berlin, Universitäts-Klinikum Steglitz,
Abteilung für Innere Medizin und Gastroenterologie,
Hindenburgdamm 30, 12203 Berlin, Germany

ZIMMER, Th.
Freie Universität Berlin, Universitäts-Klinikum Steglitz,
Abteilung für Innere Medizin und Gastroenterologie,
Hindenburgdamm 30, 12203 Berlin, Germany

# Endoscopic Fibrin Sealing in Gastroduodenal Ulcer Hemorrhage

G. HEROLD, G. PRECLIK, and E. F. STANGE

## Abstract

Patients with bleeding upper gastrointestinal ulcers were observed during the period 1989–1991. The clinical outcome was examined by retrospective analysis. Of all patients with benign gastric or duodenal ulcers, 85 patients presented with stigmata of bleeding, e.g., Forrest grades Ia–IIb. This group was treated endoscopically by the injection of fibrin sealant with or without additional hypertonic saline plus epinephrine. Endoscopic therapeutic procedures were repeated until the ulcers reached Forrest grade III. While initial hemostasis was achieved in all patients, permanent hemostasis declined to 85.9% in our series. The overall bleeding-associated mortality was 7.0%, and in 9.4% continuous bleeding required surgery. No therapy-associated complications were seen. Interestingly, fibrin glue appeared to induce a rapid healing process. It may be concluded that fibrin sealing is a complication-free highly effective endoscopic therapy.

## Introduction

Upper gastrointestinal bleeding presents a challenging problem. Endoscopy serves to evaluate bleeding of the upper gastrointestinal tract and to determine the odds of further bleeding. Several endoscopic hemostatic techniques have been advocated [1–10] in the past decade. For proper evaluation of the clinical situation and of treatment alternatives it is essential to use the Forrest classification [11, 12] as well as clinical risk factors [13]. Mortality has remained relatively constant at approximately 10%, which may be related to the increasing number of patients over 60 years old [14]. On average 20%–32% of patients suffer from continued or recurrent bleeding [14]. However, the risk may be essentially above this level in arterial spurting lesions and in ulcers with a visible vessel [15]. Endoscopic injection therapy has become an effective method of controlling and preventing nonvariceal bleeding and rebleeding [10, 16–24]. Unfortunately, all sclerosants such as polidocanol can cause tissue damage at the site of their application [25–29]. Therefore the search for effective hemostatic agents has continued. Encouraging results have been reported in the past 5 years for the injection of thrombin and fibrin sealant [30–39]. In the present work we report our experience with a fibrin sealant in a consecutive series of patients.

## Patients and Methods

A retrospective analysis of unselected patients with ulcer bleeding and subsequent endoscopic injection of fibrin sealant was performed for the period from January 1989 until December 1991. The patient data were obtained from a computerized data base [40] and subsequent analysis of the complete patient records. The patients underwent esophago-gastro-duodenoscopy within 3 following admissions. In the same session endoscopic therapy was performed, if necessary. Endoscopic controls were performed at 24-h intervals (except for rebleeding), together with recurrent injection therapy of persisting stigmata of recent hemorrhage. Spurting vessels, oozing areas, visible vessels, and adherent clots in the ulcer base were considered as stigmata according to the Forrest classification F Ia/b or F IIa/b [13, 14]. Simultaneously the patients were treated intravenously with $H_2$ receptor antagonists and since 1990 routinely with omeprazole, usually in a dose of 80 mg/day. High-risk patients were supervised in the intensive care unit.

Since 1989 we have used exclusively either the fibrin sealant (FS) alone or the combination of an initial injection of hypertonic (3.8%) saline with epinephrine 1:10000 [41] followed by the injection of fibrin sealant (HSE/FS). The fibrin sealant, Tissucol Duo S (Immuno, Heidelberg, Germany) was injected into the ulcer base as close as possible to visible vessels, blood clots, or actual bleeding areas.

During the indicated period 452 patients were seen in the Endoscopy Department with a diagnosis of one or more benign peptic ulcers: 199 (44.0%) suffered from gastric ulcers, 242 (53.5%) from duodenal ulcers, and 11 (2.4%) from stomal ulcers. The mean patient age was 58.6 years and was slightly higher in those with gastric ulcer (62.9 years) than those with duodenal ulcer (55.1 years). There were 292 men (mean age 59.8 years; 49,1% over 60) and 160 women (mean age 73.6 years; 80% over 60). A total of 85 patients (18.8%) exhibited bleeding stigmata of Forrest grades Ia–IIb and were treated with FS. The distribution of ulcers showed similar numbers for the stomach [36] and the duodenum [40], five stomal, three cardiac ulcers (sequelae of prior sclerotherapy for variceal bleeding), and one Dieulafoy ulcer. For the effective control of bleeding and stigmata of recent hemorrhage 109 therapeutic endoscopies were necessary in this group of 85 patients. At the initial endoscopy half of the ulcers (48.6%) exhibited a non-bleeding visible vessel (Forrest IIa) at the ulcer base. Of 53 visible vessels 51 had a diameter of 2 mm or less. Only a few were identified as Forrest grade Ia (5.9%), whereas 24.7% had an oozing ulcer and 23.5% an adherent clot (Forrest Ib and IIb, respectively).

In 54 endoscopies patients received FS treatment alone, and in 55 HSE/FS treatment was required to allow exact localization of the bleeding site. Seventeen patients needed more than one injection therapy to treat the bleeding stigmata and in 13 of these the twofold application was successful.

**Table 1.** Patient outcome with respect to surgery and mortality ($n = 85$)

|  | $n$ | $\%$ |
| --- | --- | --- |
| Initial success of injection therapy | 85 | 100.0 |
| Bleeding-associated surgery (rebleeding) | 8 | 9.4 |
| Bleeding-associated early elective surgery (no rebleeding) | 4 | 4.7 |
| Bleeding-independent surgery (other indications) | 2 | 2.4 |
| Bleeding-associated death after surgical intervention | 2 | 2.4 |
| Bleeding-associated mortality without surgery (rebleeding, inoperability) | 4 | 4.7 |
| Bleeding-independent death (severe basal disease, multimorbidity) | 9 | 10.6 |
| Overall bleeding-associated mortality (all patients) | 6 | 7.0 |
| Total mortality | 15 | 17.6 |
| Permanent hemostasis after therapy | 73 | 85.9 |

## *Results*

The patient outcome is described in Table 1. Eight patients needed an urgent surgical intervention because of rebleeding after primarily successful injection therapy and failure of repeated therapeutic efforts, in three of these patients. In terms of the Forrest classification these included four patients with Ia, three with Ib, and one with IIa. Early elective surgery was performed in only four patients. Two patients died of causes associated with surgery, due to multiorgan failure in one case and recurrent gastrointestinal bleeding in the other. Four patients died of bleeding-associated factors without surgical intervention (Table 1). These patients could not be operated on because of collateral disease. Due to the advanced age of many of our patients, together with concurrent illness, there were non-bleeding-related deaths in nine patients (Table 1). The overall mortality associated with upper gastrointestinal hemorrhage was 7.0 % in patients treated by endoscopic injection therapy. An overall effective hemostasis was observed in 85.9 % (Table 1).

According to the follow-up scheme 78.3 % of the patients without bleeding-associated surgery or death had a control endoscopy within 24 h after the initial endoscopic intervention. Another 14.5 % had repeat endoscopy within 48 h, and nearly all had a control within 1 week. Interestingly, in this patient group 53.6 % of the treated ulcers showed a clean, fibrin-covered ulcer base, without any bleeding stigmata between 12 and 24 h after the initial intervention, which rose to 68.1 % and 76.8 %, including the patients reendoscoped after 48 h and 3 days, respectively. It was striking that most of the fibrin-injected ulcers appeared to heal very rapidly, and that no necroses were detected in the early or late follow-up.

## Discussion

Patients in whom active bleeding or stigmata of recent hemorrhage are identified during emergency endoscopy have a high rate of rebleeding [11, 12]. We limited our intervention procedure to such patients because these findings permit an immediate therapeutic decision and are the factors influencing surgery and mortality rates [42].

Injection therapy was shown to be more effective in bleeding control than conservative management alone [16–18] and equivalent to other treatment regimens [19, 22]. A meta-analysis has indicated that all forms of endoscopic therapy appear to reduce further bleeding, surgery, and mortality rates effectively [43]. The most widely used agent for sclerotherapy is polidocanol [10] in combination with epinephrine [16, 18, 19, 20], but excellent results have also been reported for the use of epinephrine alone [17, 23]. Substantial side effects, including perforation and delayed ulcer healing [19, 25, 26, 29, 30] have been observed with polidocanol. Tissue sealing with thrombin or fibrin was introduced in the search of safer, more biocompatible agents. Alternatively, commercially available sealants may initiate coagulation within seconds, forming a submucosal fibrin clot. In an experimental study [26, 36] only minimal inflammatory reaction occurred at the site of application, no vascular thrombosis, but finally a fibroblast and collagen rich scar tissue remained.

Before 1989 primarily HSE treatment was favored, previously described by Hirao et al. [41]. However, although hypertonic saline supports the epinephrine effect by compression, the locally induced edema is short lived and bleeding recurrence is high. This regimen was therefore combined with FS to secure the bleeding site. Preinjection with HSE was used especially if active bleeding initially impaired the endoscopic overview. The additional application of omeprazole effectively blocked the gastric acidity, probably ensuring a stable thrombus formation at neutral gastric pH [44]. In other published work [32–34] the injection therapy was repeated every 24 h until the ulcer base was cleared of bleeding stigmata. The distribution of Forrest grades was similar to a previous report [34], but the number of Forrest Ia bleeders was small compared to that reported by other authors [32]. The initial hemostasis of 100 % was also achieved in other trials [32–34], including those using thrombin [36–39]. The permanent hemostasis rate of 85.9 % reported in this work is similar to that observed elsewhere [37, 39]. The observed mortality and frequency of emergency surgery is comparable to figures in the literature, ranging from 5 % to 10 % and from 5 % to 15 %, respectively [33]. Comparable results have been reported in the studies [16–20, 23] with polidocanol and/or epinephrine or epinephrine alone as well as in a small comparative study using fibrin and polidocanol [35]. A definitive comparison of the different studies and methods remains difficult due to the heterogeneous study designs, the variation in the Forrest grades of the cohort, and the applied substances.

As a consequence of the striking endoscopic results the need for surgical intervention is controversial, with reported operation frequencies varying from 0 % [34] to 51 % [21]. We also left the concept of early elective surgery if no severe rebleeding occurred and/or repeated endoscopy was successful. However, in arterial bleeders the results in terms of permanent hemostasis were disappointing, probably due to the small number. Therefore a benefit of early elective surgery in Forrest grade Ia must be examined further. Interestingly, a tendency to rapid heading, especially in the first days after therapy, was observed and seems related to FS. Although compared to other injection agents a definitive superiority of FS remains to be proven, the advantage of FS seems evident. It represents the most biological principle [45], exerts a sustained compression of the bleeding vessel, and allows a repetitive, complication-free application.

## *References*

1. Jiranek GC, Silverstein FE (1990) Introduction to endoscopic therapy for bleeding peptic ulcers. Gastrointest Endosc 36: 25–29
2. Benjamin SB (1990) Therapeutic endoscopy and bleeding ulcers: methodology. Gastrointest Endosc 36: 56–61
3. Sugawa C (1990) Injection therapy for the control of bleeding ulcers. Gastrointest Endosc 36: 50–52
4. Laine L (1990) Bipolar/multipolar electrocoagulation. Gastrointest Endosc 36: 38–41
5. Papp JP (1990) Monopolar and electrohydrothermal treatment of upper gastrointestinal bleeding. Gastrointest Endosc 36: 34–37
6. Jensen DM (1990) Heat probe for hemostasis of bleeding peptic ulcers: techniques and results of randomized controlled trials. Gastrointest Endosc 36: 42–49
7. Cotton PB (1990) Argon laser/Co$_2$ treatment of bleeding ulcers. Gastrointestinal Endosc 36: 32–33
8. Swain P (1990) Nd: YAG laser: the pro approach. Gastrointest Endosc 36: 30–31
9. Peura DA (1990) Topical therapy for the control of gastrointestinal bleeding. Gastrointest Endosc 36: 53–55
10. Soehendra N, Grimm H, Stenzel M (1985) Injection of non-variceal bleeding lesions of the upper gastrointestinal tract. Endoscopy 17: 129–132
11. Forrest JA, Finlayson NDC, Shearman DJC (1974) Endoscopy in gastrointestinal bleeding. Lancet II: 394–397
12. Heldwein WJ, Schreiner J, Pedrazzoli J, Lehnert P (1989) Is the Forrest classification a useful tool for planning endoscopic therapy of bleeding peptic ulcers? Endoscopy 21: 258–262
13. Lin H-J, Lee F-Y, Tsai Y-T, Lee S-D, Lee C-H (1990) What kind of non-bleeding visible vessel in a peptic ulcer needs aggressive therapy? Endoscopy 22: 8
14. Gilbert DA (1990) Epidemiology of upper gastrointestinal bleeding. Gastrointest Endosc 36: 8–13
15. Johnston JH (1990) Endoscopic risk factors for bleeding peptic ulcer. Gastrointest Endosc 36: 16–20
16. Panés J, Forné M, Marco C, Viver J, Garcia-Olivares E, Garau J (1987) Controlled trial of endoscopic sclerosis in bleeding peptic ulcers. Lancet 5: 1292–1294
17. Chung SCS, Leung JWC, Steele RJC, Crofts TJ, Li AKC (1988) Endoscopic injection of adrenaline for actively bleeding ulcers: a randomised trial. Br Med J 296: 1631–1633
18. Balanzó J, Sainz S, Espinós JC, Guarner C, Cussó X, Monés J, Vilardell F (1988) Endoscopic hemostasis by local injection of epinephrine and polidocanol in bleeding ulcer. A prospective randomized trial. Endoscopy 20: 289–291
19. Rutgeerts P, Broeckaert L, Janssens J, Vantrappen G, Coremans G, Hiele M (1989) Comparison of endoscopic polidocanol injection and YAG laser therapy for bleeding peptic ulcers. Lancet 27: 1164–1167

20. Panés J, Forné M, Bágena F, Viver J (1990) Endoscopic sclerosis in the treatment of bleeding peptic ulcers with a visible vessel. Am J Gastroenterol 85: 252–254
21. Winkeltau G, Arlt G, Treutner K-H, Schubert T, Schumpelick V (1990) Endoscopic therapy and early elective operation as a therapeutic regimen in ulcer bleeding. Hepatogastroenterology 37: 121–123
22. Waring JP, Sanowski RA, Sawyer RL, Woods A, Foutch PG (1991) A randomized comparison of multipolar electrocoagulation and injection sclerosis for the treatment of bleeding peptic ulcer. Gastrointest Endosc 37: 295–298
23. Steele RJC, Park KGM, Crofts TJ (1991) Adrenaline injection for endoscopic hemostasis in non-variceal upper gastrointestinal haemorrhage. Br J Surg 78: 477–479
24. Rajgopal C, Palmer KR (1991) Endoscopic injection sclerosis: effective treatment for bleeding peptic ulcer. Gut 32: 727–729
25. Rutgeerts P, Geboes P, Vantrappen G (1989) Experimental studies of injection therapy for severe nonvariceal bleedings in dogs. Gastroenterology 997: 610–621
26. Salm R, Sontheimer J, Laaff H, Cegla M (1989) Tissue reaction and hemostatic characteristics-fibrin sealant versus polidocanol: experimental and clinical results. In: Waclawiczek HW (ed) Progress in fibrin sealing. Springer, Berlin Heidelberg New York, pp 123–129
27. Levy J, Khakoo S, Barton R, Vicary R (1991) Fatal injection sclerotherapy of a bleeding peptic ulcer. Lancet 337: 504
28. Chester JF, Hurley PR (1990) Gastric necrosis: a complication of endoscopic sclerosis for bleeding peptic ulcer. Endoscopy 22: 287
29. Loperfido S, Patelli G, La Torre L (1990) Extensive necrosis of gastric mucosa following injection therapy of bleeding peptic ulcer. Endoscopy 22: 285–286
30. Eimiller A (1988) Fibrinkleber als Sklerosierungsmittel bei blutenden Läsionen im Gastrointestinaltrakt. In: Manegold BC (ed) Fibrinklebung in der Endoskopie. Springer, Berlin Heidelberg New York, pp 79–84
31. Groitl H, Scheele J (1987) Initial experience with the endoscopic application of fibrin tissue adhesive in the upper gastrointestinal tract. Surg Endosc 1: 93–97
32. Salm R, Sontheimer J, Cegla M, Rückauer K (1989) Endoskopische Fibrinkleber-Injektion zur Blutstillung beim peptischen Ulcus. Endoskopie Heute 3: 63–66
33. Friedrichs O, Beccu L, Knieriem H-J, Papen J, Sabinasz A (1990) Submucöse Fibrinklebung bei peptischen Blutungen. In: Häring R (ed) Gastrointestinale Blutung. Blackwell Ueberreuter, Berlin, pp 101–108
34. Friedrichs O, Papen J, Sabinasz A, Heppe M (1990) Submucöse Fibrinklebung der Ulcusblutung – hat sich das Konzept bewährt? Z Gastroenterol 28: 477 (abstract)
35. Prassler R, Hendrich H, Richter G, Barnert J, Wienbeck M (1991) Endoskopische Therapie mit Polidocanol und Fibrinkleber bei der akuten Ulcusblutung. Z Gastroenterol 29: 491 (abstract)
36. Fuchs K-H, Schaube H, Hamelmann H (1990). Die endoskopische Blutstillung mit der Injektionsmethode. In: Häring R (ed) Gastrointestinale Blutung. Blackwell Ueberreuter, Berlin, pp 89–96
37. Balanzó J, Villanueva C, Sainz S, Espinós JC, Mendez C, Guarner C, Vilardell F (1990) Injection therapy of bleeding peptic ulcer. A prospective, randomized trial using epinephrine and thrombin. Endoscopy 22: 157–159
38. Fuchs K-H, Schaube H, Eckstein AK, Freys S (1989) Die endoskopische Hämostase. In: Henning H, Manegold BC (eds) Fortschritte der gastroenterologischen Endoskopie, vol 19. Demeter, Gräfelfing, pp 88–93
39. Benedetti G, Sablich R, Lacchin T (1991) Endoscopic injection sclerotherapy in nonvariceal upper gastrointestinal bleeding. Surg Endosc 5: 28–30
40. Swobodnik W, Kuhn K (1992) Elektronische Befunddokumentation, Leistungsstatistik und Bildanalysen in der Endoskopie. Z Gastroenterol 30: 202–203
41. Hirao M, Kobayashi T, Masuda K, Yamaguchi S, Noda K, Matsuura K, Naka H, Kawauchi H, Namiki M (1985) Endoscopic local injection of hypertonic saline-epinephrine solution to arrest hemorrhage from the upper gastrointestinal tract. Gastrointest Endosc 31: 313–317

42. Sarkar MR, Kienzle H-F, Bähr R (1992) Kann durch endoskopische Methoden die Letalitäts- und Komplikationsrate des blutenden Ulcus ventriculi bzw. duodeni gesenkt werden? Leber Magen Darm 1: 10–18
43. Cook DJ, Guyatt GH, Salena BJ, Laine LA (1992) Endoscopic therapy for acute nonvariceal upper gastrointestinal hemorrhage: a metaanalysis. Gastroenterology 102: 139–148
44. Brunner G, Chang J (1990) Intravenous therapy with high doses of ranitidine and omeprazole in critically ill patients with bleeding peptic ulcerations of the upper intestinal tract: an open randomized controlled trial. Digestion 45: 217–225
45. Manegold BC (1988) Endoskopische Fibrinklebung. Endoskopie Heute 2: 22–24

# Endoscopic Injection Therapy of Gastroduodenal Ulcer Hemorrhage: A Randomized Comparison of Fibrin Sealant vs. Polidocanol

R. SALM, K. E. GRUND, J. SONTHEIMER, A. BUSTOS, and E. WEBER

## Abstract

In a randomized trial involving 56 patients with acute gastroduodenal ulcer hemorrhage we examined the rebleeding rate after endoscopic local injection of fibrin sealant (group A, $n = 30$) in comparison to polidocanol (group B, $n = 26$). Included were ulcers with spurting (Forrest Ia) or oozing bleeding (F Ib) or a visible vessel (F IIa). In case of F Ia/Ib the endoscopic therapy in both groups was combined with a preliminary injection of epinephrine ($1:10^4$). After endoscopic hemostasis the patients were transferred to the surgical intensive care unit. The patients underwent routine endoscopy 24 h later. If rebleeding signs occurred, emergency endoscopy was performed. In the case of rebleeding or a still visible vessel another injection therapy now with fibrin sealant in both groups was performed. Initial hemostasis was achieved in 100% of cases in group A and in 77% in group B ($p \leq 0.05$). Recurrent hemorrhage occurred in 10% in group A and in 38% in group B ($p \leq 0.05$). Permanent hemostasis was achieved in 93% in group A and 88% in group B. There were no differences between the two groups in the requirement for emergency surgery or mortality. A tendency toward a lower blood transfusion requirement was observed in group A, but it failed to achieve statistical significance. No complications of injection therapy were noted.

## Introduction

Progress in therapy of gastroduodenal ulcer bleeding is based on endoscopic diagnosis and endoscopic hemostasis. The value of endoscopic hemostasis has been demonstrated by a meta-analysis of controlled studies with respect to the end-points further bleeding, surgery, and mortality [4]. Advantages were revealed for patients with endoscopic signs of bleeding risk, i.e., with active hemorrhage or nonbleeding visible vessel. The most frequently employed endoscopic hemostasis methods are the application of thermal energy (e.g., electrocoagulation, electro-hydro-thermal probe, laser coagulation) or the local injection of epinephrine or sclerosing agents. Injection therapy has become a popular method because it is simple, safe, and inexpensive [6]. Injection therapy acts mainly as a tamponade in the initial phase of hemostasis. Using epinephrine provides additional vasoconstriction [3].

Both thermal or sclerosing methods cause tissue injury and prolonged healing; a perforation may even result [5, 18]. As we know from endoscopic sclerosing therapy of esophageal varices tissue damage can also induce rebleeding [22]. In the case of gastroduodenal ulcer bleeding tissue destruction or delay of the healing process should be avoided because only the healed ulcer prevents rebleeding. Therefore it seems to be logical to use fibrin sealant instead of sclerosing agents in gastroduodenal ulcer hemorrhage; fibrin sealant causes no tissue damage and has additional effects on hemostasis and wound healing. In a prospective uncontrolled trial we confirmed the feasibility and effectiveness of endoscopic injection therapy with fibrin sealant in gastroduodenal ulcer bleeding [21]. Afterwards we started a randomized controlled study comparing fibrin sealant with polidocanol.

## Patients and Methods

The study was carried out at the Department of General Surgery, University Hospital Freiburg, and the Department of General Surgery, University Hospital Tübingen. Included were patients with gastroduodenal ulcer bleeding, Forrest (F) classification F Ia (spurting), F Ib (oozing) or F IIa (visible vessel) [9]. Verification of visible vessels with Doppler sonography was on the basis of arterial noise in less than 1 mm depth. Exclusion criteria were: pregnancy, age under 18 years, preexisting disorder of blood coagulation, preceding endoscopic treatment before admission in our hospital, and impossibility of endoscopic therapy (e.g. insufficient visibility, hemodynamic instability). Initial emergency endoscopy was performed immediately after emergency measures, using the Olympus endoscopes: GIF 1T10, GIF 2T10 (Olympus Optical, Hamburg). All patients undergoing emergency endoscopy for bleeding gave informed consent for possible endoscopic hemostasis therapy; the treatment option group A (fibrin sealant) or group B (polidocanol) was in a sealed envelope.

In the case of F Ia or Ib stage we first injected epinephrine (Suprarenin, Hoechst, Frankfurt; dilution: $1:10^4$, max. 1 mg) into the ulcer base in both groups; after randomization the measure was completed with injection of either fibrin sealant (group A; Tissucol Duo S, human fibrinogen, human thrombin, steam treated, Immuno, Heidelberg) or polidocanol (group B, Aethoxysklerol Kreussler 1%, Kreussler, Wiesbaden). After normal endoscopy all patients were transferred to the surgical intensive care unit. The patients were given intravenous omeprazol (initially 80 mg, then 40 mg/8 h), transfusion of erythrocyte concentrates, and fresh plasma, if necessary. All patients underwent programmed endoscopic control after 24 h or on emergency basis at clinical signs of recurrent hemorrhage; further controls were carried out 3 and 7 days after the last hemostasis treatment.

Clinical signs of rebleeding were: reappearance of hematemesis, tarry or bloody stools, renewed tachycardia (pulse > 100 beats/min) or hypotension (systolic blood pressure < 100 mgHg) after primary stabilization. Repeated injection therapy was carried out in the case of F Ia, Ib, or IIa at time of reendoscopy. In contrast to the primary hemostasis method fibrin sealant was used in both groups. The reason for changing the injection agent to fibrin sealant in the polidocanol group was the perforation risk with repeated injection of sclerosing agents. Emergency surgery was performed in the case of failure of primary or repeated endoscopic hemostasis measure. Failure of endoscopic hemostasis was assumed if bleeding did not stop after injection of a total amount of 20 ml of the respective substance (polidocanol or fibrin sealant) and additional epinephrine (1 mg max.). After thawing, which takes about 3–5 min, the two components of the fibrin sealant were either injected simultaneously through a double-lumen cannula or consecutively through a single-lumen cannula: first fibrinogen and then thrombin. Between these, the single-lumen cannula was rinsed with physiological sodium chloride solution. The cannula was pierced vertically or slightly tangentially in several positions (generally four to six times) around and in the bleeding source. By slowly retracting the cannula approx. 0.5 ml of the substance was injected each time.

The sample size was calculated as 88 patients per group. This was based on a rate of recurrent bleeding of about 23 % using polidocanol and an estimated decrease by 50 % using fibrin sealant [14, 16, 20, 23]. Type I/II error were fixed at 10 % and 20 %, respectively. Statistical analysis was performed using Fisher's exact test. A probability value of $p \leq 0.05$ was considered significant.

The investigation was initiated in autumn of 1990. Because of the result of the first planned interim evaluation, which proved an advantage of fibrin sealant over polidocanol, the study was terminated in July 1992. At this time 56 patients had been included, 30 in group A and 26 in group B. Only three patients hat to be excluded: two had previous endoscopic therapy in another hospital, and one suffered from preexisting disorder of blood coagulation. The average age of the two groups was comparable (group A, 62.7 ± 18.2 years; group B, 58.0 ± 16.8 years). Women were significantly underrepresented in group B (4/26), whereas in group A nearly half of the patients were women (14/30). The distribution of ulcer location was comparable in the two groups (Table 1). Bleeding activity was slightly less favorable in group A.

**Table 1.** Ulcer location and bleeding activity (UV = ulcer ventriculi; UD = ulcer duodeni), ($n = 56$)

| Forrest stage | Group A | | Group B | | Total | |
|---|---|---|---|---|---|---|
| | UV | UD | UV | UD | UV | UD |
| Ia | 4 | 6 | 2 | 1 | 6 | 7 |
| Ib | 3 | 4 | 4 | 5 | 7 | 9 |
| IIa | 5 | 8 | 7 | 7 | 12 | 15 |
| Total | 12 | 18 | 13 | 13 | 25 | 31 |

UV, Ulcer ventriculi; UD, ulcer duodeni.

## Results

Initially, all active hemorrhages were stopped endoscopically in group A. In two patients with F IIa stage in this group hemorrhage was initiated by injection, which stopped after further injection. In four patients of group B, the bleeding recurred during emergency endoscopy after initial hemostasis. It increased despite further injection and could not be stopped with the predetermined volume of polidocanol or epinephrine. For these four patients fibrin sealant was applied in addition instead of performing emergency surgery. This procedure was successful in all cases, in the further course no recurrent hemorrhage was observed.

Recurrent hemorrhages were seen in 3 of 30 patients (10%) in group A and in 10 of 26 patients (38%) in group B ($p \leq 0.05$). All recurrences were observed during the first 72 h. By means of additional injection therapy with fibrin sealant a permanent endoscopic hemostasis was achieved in 28 of 30 cases (93%) in group A and in 23 of 26 cases (88%) in group B (Table 2). No statistical difference was observed in the need for emergency surgery in the two groups (two cases in group A and three in group B) (Table 2). Five patients died (three in group A, two in group B) without a relapse of bleeding. None of the operated patients died. The causes of death were decompensated heart failure and advanced stage of malignoma.

On average 5.1 ml fibrin sealant (both components together) was used in group A for initial and repeated injection therapy. In group B the average injection volume of polidocanol was 12.4 ml polidocanol and another 2.9 ml fibrin sealant in cases of insufficient hemostasis or relapse. The number of blood transfusions showed no difference between the groups. Taking only the patients from the two groups in which the endoscopic injection therapy was successful without emergency surgery the following relation was determined: patients in group A received on average $4.3 \pm 2.1$ U and those in group B $6.1 \pm 3.6$ U erythrocyte concentrates. This difference was statistically not significant. In two patients an increasing ulcer area was observed after polidocanol injection. No complications after endoscopic injection of fibrin sealant were noted.

**Table 2.** Clinical course after endoscopic injection therapy ($n = 56$)

| Forrest stage | n | | Recurrent hemorrhage | | Permanent endoscopic hemostasis | | Surgery to control bleeding | | Mortality | |
|---|---|---|---|---|---|---|---|---|---|---|
| | A | B | A | B | A | B | A | B | A | B |
| Ia | 10 | 3 | 2 | 3 | 9 | 3 | 1 | – | 1 | – |
| Ib | 7 | 9 | – | 2 | 7 | 8 | – | 1 | – | – |
| IIa | 13 | 14 | 1 | 5 | 12 | 12 | 1 | 2 | 2 | 2 |
| Total | 30 | 26 | 3* | 10* | 28 | 23 | 2 | 3 | 3 | 2 |

* $p \leq 0.05$.

## Discussion

One of the most commonly used procedures in the emergency treatment of bleeding peptic ulcers is the endoscopic injection therapy of sclerotherapeutics and/or epinephrine. The application of sclerosing agents causes significant tissue injury, which can retard the ulcer healing process [13]. This could be a negative factor influencing the rebleeding rate. Fibrin sealant has been successfully applied in operative medicine for hemostatic purpose for several years. Tissue-destroying effects are not to be expected using this substance. However, limited experience of endoscopic hemostatic measures with fibrin sealant is available [7, 8, 10, 11, 21]. Therefore, we compared in a randomized trial the efficacy of fibrin sealant with that of polidocanol in 56 patients with acute peptic ulcer hemorrhage. The agents were endoscopically injected in the bleeding source. The main criterion was the relapse rate. Only actively bleeding ulcers or those with a visible vessel were included, because there is a high risk for rebleeding [12, 26].

These data and the bleeding activity correspond to epidemiological data [1, 15, 19]. In our series active hemorrhage stages (Forrest Ia/Ib) were slightly more frequent in the group treated with fibrin sealant. Especially the F Ia type predominated compared to the polidocanol group. It is conspicuous that the number or recurrent hemorrhages of the ulcers treated with fibrin sealant was only one-third of the polidocanol treated ones. Noticable are also the ulcers with a visible vessel but which do not bleed at the time of endoscopy: in the polidocanol group about one-third of the patients had recurrent hemorrhages whereas in the fibrin sealant group this occurred in only one-tenth. However, there was no advantage concerning the frequency of surgery (10 % vs. 7.7 %). This may be due to the fact that in cases of failure or relapse in the polidocanol group there was an attempt with injection of fibrin sealant. Thereby emergency surgery could be avoided in at least four patients. On the other hand, the observed high relapse rate in the polidocanol group seems to be realistic; a recently published study with 33 patients showed a rebleeding rate of only 22 % after injection therapy with epinephrine plus polidocanol [25]. But in this group there were no spurting bleeding ulcers, only oozing or nonbleeding visible vessels. The overall mortality rate was 8.9 %, with no difference between the groups. None of the operated patients died. None of the deceased patients had suffered from relapse.

Until now there have been two randomized studies comparing fibrin sealant with polidocanol and another one with a historical control. A historical comparative study was published by Prassler et al. [17]. In a 2-year period 100 patients were treated with laser therapy, bipolar electrocoagulation, or polidocanol injection. In the following year injection therapy with fibrin sealant was performed in 60 patients with ulcer hemorrhage. The definitive hemostasis ratio in the fibrin sealant series was significantly higher ($p \leq 0.05$) than in the historical series. Operation frequency and mortality were reduced. Berg et al. achieved results similar to those of our study [2]. However, they also treated F IIb ulcers; as a conclusion they report a more effective reduction of recurrence rate after fibrin sealant than with polidocanol. A statistical evaluation was not presented. Strohm et al. treated 60 patients with ulcer hemorrhage [24]. On a randomized basis the ulcers of 29 patients were injected with fibrin sealant and in 31 cases adrenaline or polidocanol was injected or electro-coagulation therapy was performed (APE). Eight recurrent hemorrhages occurred in the fibrin sealant group as opposed to seven after APE application. Two patients belonging to the APE group died. An advantage of fibrin sealant therapy was not observed. The reason for this can possibly lie in the imbalance of 5 to 0 arterial hemorrhages in the fibrin sealant and APE groups.

We conclude that the endoscopic injection of fibrin sealant for acute ulcer hemorrhage is feasible and effective. Our study showed a significant advantage in the fibrin sealant group with respect to the principal criterion of "recurrent hemorrhage." The prerequisite of successful endoscopic hemostasis with fibrin sealant, however, is control of the application technique, which requires training for the endoscopist and his team.

## References

1. Balanzó J, Sáinz S, Such J, Espinós JC, Guarner C, Cussó X, Monés J, Vilardell F (1988) Endoscopic hemostasis by local injection of epinephrine and polidocanol in bleeding ulcer. A prospective randomized trial. Endoscopy 20: 289–291
2. Berg P, Barina W, Born P, Simon W, Zellmer R, Paul F (1990) Fibrinkleber versus Polidocanol bei der oberen Gastrointestinalblutung. In: Henning H, Soehendra N (eds) Fortschritte der gastroenterologischen Endoskopie. Demeter, Gräfelfing, pp 22–24
3. Chung SC, Leung FW, Leung JW (1988) Is vasoconstriction the mechanism of hemostasis in bleeding ulcers injected with epinephrine? A study using reflectance spectrophotometry. Gastrointest Endosc 34: 174–175
4. Cook DJ, Guyatt GH, Salena BJ, Laine LA (1992) Endoscopic therapy for acute nonvariceal gastrointestinal hemorrhage: a meta-analysis. Gastroenterology 102: 139–148
5. Dennis MB, Peoples J, Hulett R, Auth DC, Protell RL, Rubin CE, Silverstein FE (1979) Evaluation of electrofulguration in control of bleeding of experimental gastric ulcers. Dig Dis Sci 24: 845–848
6. Eastwood GL (1992) Endoscopy in gastrointestinal bleeding. Are we beginning to realize the dream? J Clin Gastroenterol 14: 187–191
7. Eimiller A (1988) Fibrinkleber als Sklerosierungsmittel. In: Manegold BC (ed) Fibrinklebung in der Endoskopie. Springer, Berlin Heidelberg New York, pp 79–84
8. Friedrichs O (1991) Submucöse Fibrinklebung der akuten Ulkusblutung – hat sich das Konzept bewährt? Intensiv Notfallbehandl 16: 163–168
9. Forrest JA, Finlayson ND, Shearman DJ (1974) Endoscopy in gastrointestinal bleeding. Lancet II: 394–397
10. Fuchs KH, Wirtz HJ, Schaube H (1992) Endoskopisch-chirurgische Blutstillung im Gastrointestinaltrakt. In: Fuchs KH, Manegold BC (eds) Chirurgische Endoskopie im Abdomen. Blackwell Wissenschaft, Berlin, pp 47–69
11. Grund KE, Mohl W, Fischer H (1991) Endoskopische Fibrinklebung – Indikation, Ergebnisse und Probleme. Endoskopie Heute 4: 53–54
12. Johnston JH (1990) Endoscopic risk factors for bleeding peptic ulcer. Gastrointest Endosc 36: S16–S20
13. Kalabakas A, Swain CP (1992) A comparison of injection and topical application of fibrin tissue glue with injection and thermal methods for the treatment of standard experimental bleeding ulcers. Endoscopy 24: 616–617

14. Kortan P, Haber G, Marcon N (1986) Endoscopic injection therapy for nonvariceal lesions of the upper gastrointestinal tract. Gastrointest Endosc 32: 145
15. Laine L (1990) Multipolar electrocoagulation versus injection therapy in the treatment of bleeding peptic ulcers. Gastroenterology 99: 1303–1306
16. Panés J, Viver J, Forné M, Garcia-Olivares E, Marco C, Garau J (1987) Controlled trial of endoscopic sclerosis in bleeding peptic ulcers. Lancet II: 1292–1294
17. Prassler R, Barnert J, Richter G, Wienbeck M (1992) Die endoskopische Fibrinklebung bei blutenden Magen- und Duodenalulzera. Intensiv Notfallbehandl 17: 43–47
18. Randall GM, Jensen DM, Hirabayashi K, Machicado GA (1989) Controlled study of different sclerosing agents for coagulation of canine gut arteries. Gastroenterology 96: 1274–1281
19. Roggo A, Filippini L (1990) Endoskopische Injektionstherapie bei akuter nichtvariköser oberer Gastrointestinalblutung. Dtsch Med Wochenschr 115: 1227–1231
20. Rutgeerts P, Gevers AM, Hiele M, Broeckaert L, Coremans G, Janssens J, Vantrappen G (1990) Injection therapy for prevention of rebleeding from peptic ulcers with protruding vessel: which method is best? Gastroenterology 98: A115
21. Salm R, Bohle W, Sontheimer J (1991) Peptic ulcer hemorrhage: Local injection of fibrin sealant – experimental and clinical data. Acta Chir Austr 23: 113–116
22. Siemens F, Paquet KJ, Koussouris P, Mercado MA, Kalk JF (1989) Long-term endoscopic injection sclerotherapy of bleeding esophageal varices. A prospective analysis of results by endoscopy, manometry and 24-h pH-monitoring. Surg Endosc 3: 137–141
23. Soehendra N, Grimm H, Stenzel M (1985) Injection of nonvariceal bleeding lesions of the upper gastrointestinal tract. Endoscopy 17: 129–132
24. Strohm WD, Römmele U, Barton E, Paul-Martin C (1994) Injektionstherapie des blutenden Ulcus pepticum mit Fibrin oder Polidocanol. Dtsch Med Wschr 119: 249–256
25. Villanueva C, Balanzó J, Espinós JC, Fábrega E, Sáinz S, Gonzáles D, Vilardell F (1993) Endoscopic injection therapy of bleeding ulcer: a prospective and randomized comparison of adrenaline alone or with polidocanol. J Clin Gastroenterol 17: 195–200
26. Wara P (1985) Endoscopic prediction of major rebleeding – a prospective study of stigmata of hemorrhage in bleeding ulcer. Gastroenterology 88: 1209–1214

# Submucosal Fibrin Adhesion in Upper Gastrointestinal Bleeding

J. Labenz, U. Peitz, M. Wieczorek, and G. Börsch

## Abstract

During the past 15 years, several methods of endoscopic hemostasis have been evaluated in clinical studies for injection therapy with adrenaline/polidocanol. However, these substances may produce tissue damage. In some pilot studies, excellent results concerning initial and definitive control of peptic ulcer hemorrhage were obtained with submucosal injection of a fibrin tissue adhesive.

In the past 2½ years, 83 patients with upper gastrointestinal (GI) bleeding – peptic ulcer hemorrhage, $n = 68$ (Forrest I a, $n = 16$; I b, $n = 20$; II a, $n = 29$; II b, $n = 3$); Mallory-Weiss tear, $n = 3$; varices, $n = 3$; esophageal ulcer/esophagitis, $n = 4$; angiodysplasia, $n = 2$; gastric carcinoma, $n = 1$; and sphincterotomy bleeding, $n = 2$ – diagnosed endoscopically were treated with a two-component fibrin adhesive (Tissucol Duo S, Immuno, Heidelberg, Germany) via a double lumen catheter. Initial control of bleeding was achieved in 96.4% (80/83) of patients. Early rebleeding occurred in 11 out of 80 patients (13.8%), which could be effectively managed by repeated injection of the fibrin adhesive in six patients. Nine patients (10.8%) required emergency ($n = 5$) or elective surgery ($n = 4$). The overall mortality rate was 6.0%. Complications due to submucosal injection of the fibrin adhesive were not observed.

*In conclusion*, endoscopic submucosal injection of a fibrin adhesive was highly effective (96.4% of patients) in initial control of upper GI hemorrhage predominantly due to peptic ulcer bleeding. By including repeated injections, definitive hemostasis was achieved in 90.4%. Prospective, randomized, and controlled studies are necessary to confirm these encouraging results.

## Introduction

During the past 15 years, several methods for endoscopic treatment of gastrointestinal bleeding (GI), have been evaluated in clinical studies and proved to be highly successful with regard to initial control of bleeding and reduction of bleeding relapses, frequency of surgical interventions, and mortality [3]. The hemostatic mechanisms included local edema and reduction of blood flow induced by vasoconstrictives and thermic (electro- and laser-coagulation, heater probe) or chemical lesions (e.g., polidocanol) of the tissue [8].

Most endoscopists now prefer sclerotherapy, because this method is easy to learn, practicable everywhere, cheap, and of equal efficiency compared with the other methods mentioned above. However, the injected sclerosants produce tissue damage, entailing the risk of rebleeding and severe complications [2, 7].

Fibrin sealant seems to be a suitable substance for transendoscopic injection therapy, because it combines efficient initial hemostasis and the first step of wound healing (substrate phase) without additional damage to tissue. Fibrin sealant was superior to polidocanol in experimental studies with Wistar rats [8], and excellent results concerning initial and definitive hemostasis were obtained in some pilot studies in humans with upper GI bleeding predominantly due to peptic ulcer hemorrhage [4, 6, 8].

## Patients and Methods

In the past 3 years, 100 patients with upper GI bleeding of various etiology were endoscopically treated with submucosal or intravariceal injection of 1–2 ml of a two-component fibrin tissue adhesive (Tissucol Duo S, Immuno, Heidelberg, Germany) via a double lumen catheter. In some patients with active peptic ulcer bleeding or visible vessel, 4–10 ml adrenaline (1:10000) was additionally injected in the surroundings of the bleeding lesion. All patients also received omeprazole or ranitidine intravenously. Re-endoscopies were performed within the next 24 h or when recurrent bleeding was suspected clinically. Lesions with active rebleeding or visible vessel were again treated as described above.

## Results

The indications for submucosal fibrin adhesion comprised bleeding from peptic ulcers ($n = 80$), Mallory-Weiss tears ($n = 6$), esophageal ulcers/esophagitis ($n = 5$), angiodysplasias ($n = 3$), esophageal, fundic, and duodenal varices ($n = 3$), sphincterotomy wound ($n = 2$), and gastric carcinoma ($n = 1$). An overview of treatment results is given in Table 1.

Initial hemostasis was achieved in all but one patient with active bleeding from duodenal or gastric ulcers ($n = 41$). In one patient with arterial bleeding from an ulcer at the posterior wall of the duodenal bulb, injection therapy failed to induce hemostasis. A bleeding relapse was observed in 12 patients with peptic ulcers, which was effectively managed by repeated injections of fibrin sealant in seven patients. Emergency ($n = 5$) or early elective surgery ($n = 3$) was done in eight patients (Table 2).

Hemostasis without evidence of a bleeding relapse was achieved in all patients with hemorrhage due to Mallory-Weiss tear, esophageal ulcer or esophagitis, and angiodysplasia. Intravascular injection of fibrin adhesive primarily

**Table 1.** Overview of clinical results of endoscopic hemostasis by injection of fibrin sealant in 100 patients

|  | Number of patients | Percentage |
|---|---|---|
| Initial success of fibrin sealant | 97/100 | 97 |
| Recurrent bleeding | 14/ 97 | 14.4 |
| Definitive hemostasis by fibrin sealant | 87/100 | 87 |
| Sclerotherapy with polidocanol or histoacryl | 3/100 | 3 |
| Emergency surgery | 6/100 | 6 |
| Early elective surgery | 3/100 | 3 |
| Elective surgery | 1/100 | 1 |
| Mortality (30 days) | 6/100 | 6 |

failed in two patients with esophageal and fundic variceal hemorrhage, respectively. A bleeding relapse from a duodenal varix several days after successful control with fibrin sealant was definitely cured by endoscopic embolization with Histoacryl (Braun-Melsungen). In one of two patients with arterial postsphincterotomy bleeding, emergency surgery was required. Arterial bleeding from a gastric carcinoma induced by forceps biopsy stopped after intratumor application of fibrin sealant. This patient was electively operated after the routine staging procedure (Table 3).The overall mortality within 30 days was six out of 100 (6%). In four cases, deaths were closely related to the upper GI bleeding, whereas two patients died from a cardiac insufficiency and cerebral apoplexia, respectively. Local or systemic side effects due to the endoscopic application of the fibrin tissue adhesive were not observed.

**Table 2.** Overview of clinical results of endoscopic hemostasis by injection of fibrin sealant in 80 patients with peptic ulcer hemorrhage

|  | Stage of bleeding[a] | | | | Total | |
|---|---|---|---|---|---|---|
|  | Ia | Ib | IIa | IIb | (n) | (%) |
| Initial success of fibrin sealant | 18/19 | 22/22 | 36/36 | 3/ 3 | 79/80 | 98.8 |
| Recurrent bleeding | 4/18 | 1/22 | 6/36 | 1/ 3 | 12/79 | 15.2 |
| Definitive hemostasis | 15/19 | 22/22 | 33/36 | 2/ 3 | 72/80 | 90.0 |
| Surgery | 4/19 | 0/22 | 3/36 | 1/ 3 | 8/80 | 10.0 |
| Mortality (30 days) | 1/19 | 1/22 | 3/36 | 0/22 | 5/80 | 6.25 |

[a] Categories according to the Forrest classification [5].

**Table 3.** Overview of clinical results of endoscopic hemostasis by injection of fibrin sealant in 20 patients with nonulcer hemorrhage in the upper gastrointestinal tract

|  | Initial success | Rebleeding | Definitive treatment | Mortality |
|---|---|---|---|---|
| Mallory-Weiss tear | 6/6 | 0 | – | 0/6 |
| Esophageal ulcer/esophagitis | 5/5 | 0 | – | 0/5 |
| Varices: |  |  |  |  |
|   Esophageal | 0/1 | – | Polidocanol | 0/1 |
|   Fundic | 0/1 | – | Histoacryl | 0/1 |
|   Duodenal | 1/1 | 1/1 | Histoacryl | 0/1 |
| Angiodysplasia | 3/3 | 0 | – | 0/3 |
| Sphincterotomy bleeding | 2/2 | 1/2 | Surgery | 1/2 |
| Gastric carcinoma | 1/1 | 0 | Surgery | 0/1 |

## Discussion

The results presented here clearly demonstrate that transendoscopic submucosal injection of a fibrin tissue sealant via a double lumen catheter is an efficacious and safe method to treat various bleeding lesions in the upper GI tract. We obtained fairly high rates of initial and definitive hemostasis in patients with nonvariceal bleeding. The data are in accordance with those reported by other authors [1, 4, 6, 8]. However, these encouraging results still have to be definitively confirmed by prospective, randomized, and controlled studies. A first attempt done by Strohm and coworkers in a small-scale randomized trial failed to demonstrate a statistically significant superiority of fibrin sealant over conventional sclerotherapy with adrenaline and polidocanol [9]. Therefore, the recommendation of a routine use of fibrin sealant for endoscopic sclerotherapy of bleeding lesions in the upper GI tract is presently based on the theoretical advantage of this physiological substance (avoidance of additional tissue damage, first step of wound healing), the results obtained in animal experiments in rats, and the experience of several investigators in large, but uncontrolled, studies.

## Conclusions

Endoscopic submucosal injection of a fibrin tissue adhesive proved to be highly successful concerning initial and definitive control of upper GI bleeding predominantly due to peptic ulcers in an uncontrolled series of 100 patients. Local or systemic side effects were not observed. This clearly suggests fibrin sealant as a suitable substance for endoscopic sclerotherapy and as a highly valuable addition to the endotherapeutic armamentarium. However, before this therapeutic strategy can be recommended as the routine method of choice with any superiority compared to previous means of inducing hemostasis in GI bleeding, the results of further randomized and controlled studies have to be awaited.

## References

1. Berg P, Born P, Barina W, Simon W, Zellmer R, Paul F (1990) Fibrinkleber versus Polidocanol bei der oberen Gastrointestinalblutung. Z Gastroenterol 28: 467
2. Chester JF, Hurley PR (1990) Gastric necrosis: a complication of endoscopic sclerosis for bleeding peptic ulcers. Endoscopy 22: 287
3. Cook DJ, Guyatt GH, Salena BJ, Laine LA (1992) Endoscopic therapy for acute nonvariceal upper gastrointestinal hemorrhage: a meta-analysis. Gastroenterology 102: 139–148
4. Eimiller A, Berg P, Bor P, Barina W, Paul F, Homann H (1989) A new development in gastrointestinal bleeding: sclerotherapy using a fibrin sealant. In: Waclawiczek HW (ed) Progress in fibrin sealing. Springer, Berlin Heidelberg New York, pp 131–134
5. Forrest JAM, Finlayson NDC, Shearmen DJC (1974) Endoscopy in gastrointestinal bleeding. Lancet II: 394–397
6. Friedrichs O (1992) Submucosal fibrin adhesion in peptic ulcer bleeding. Hellenic J Gastroenterol 5 [Suppl]: 86
7. Loperfido S, Patelli G, La Torre L (1990) Extensive necrosis of gastric mucosa following injection therapy of bleeding peptic ulcer. Endoscopy 22: 285–286
8. Salm R, Sontheimer J, Laaff H, Cegla M (1989) Tissue reaction and hemostatic characteristics – fibrin sealant versus polidocanol: experimental and clinical results. In: Waclawiczek HW (ed) Progress in fibrin sealing. Springer, Berlin Heidelberg New York, pp 123–129
9. Strohm WD, Römmele UE, Barton E, Weimer J (1992) Fibrinklebung und konventionelle Injektionstherapie bei blutenden Ulzera im oberen GI-Trakt. Z Gastroenterol 30: 687

# Laparoscopic Surgical Treatment of Duodenal Ulcer Disease

J. Mouiel, N. Katkhouda, and L. Iovine

## Abstract

Laparoscopic surgical treatment of duodenal ulcer disease is as safe and efficient as in open surgery and the usefulness of fibrin sealing had been demonstrated in elective cases and in emergency. In elective cases posterior truncal vagotomy and seromyotomy according the Taylor's procedure were used in 62 patients resistant to medical treatment and noncompliant to maintenance drugs. In all cases seromyotomy was closed by an overlap running suture secured by application of fibrin sealant. In emergency cases a laparoscopic approach was performed for perforated ulcer in 28 patients: after complete peritoneal toilet and closure of the perforation with an omental flap fibrin sealing completed the approximation of tissues. The follow-up was uneventful in 27 patients, and one death observed in an ASA III patient converted to open surgery due to duodenal wall lesions and delay of operation. In laparoscopic surgery the use of fibrin sealing is helpful and efficient to complete hemostasis and secure sutures.

## Introduction

Laparoscopic surgical treatment of duodenal ulcer disease is currently performed routinely [8–12] thanks to the experience gained in basic procedures both in elective cases resistant to medical treatment by posterior vagotomy and anterior seromyotomy, as described by Taylor [16], in emergency for perforated ulcer by suture of the ulcer associated with omental flap. In these two indications the use of fibrin sealing is helpful and efficient.

## Principle of the Operation

The principle of the elective operation is based on the anatomical studies of Latarjet, who showed that the secretory nerves, originating from the anterior and posterior gastric nerves, course through the superficial seromuscular layer of the stomach before penetrating the gastric wall beyond the vascular pedicles. Division of the seromuscular layer only, sparing the inner mucosa, interrupts the secretory branches of the vagus nerves. It has been established experimentally that to be efficacious seromyotomy should be performed precisely 1.5 cm from and parallel to the lesser curvature. In his original technique described in 1979 [16], Taylor advocated incision of the seromuscular layer of the anterior and posterior aspects of the stomach beginning at the incisura cardiaca and continuing to the incisura angularis which, in reality, corresponds to fundic denervation. In 1982 [17] Taylor et al. proposed replacing posterior seromyotomy by posterior truncal vagotomy as Hill and Barker had already advocated in 1978 for highly selective vagotomy [5]. Complete division of the posterior vagus nerve ensures total denervation of the posterior parasympathetic territory without creating any adverse secondary effects on the pancreas or the digestive tracts, as shown by Smith [15] and Burge [1]. This means that there is no secondary postoperative diarrhea, and that antropyloric motility is preserved.

Indeed, as anterior seromyotomy preserves the antropyloric seromyotomy branches of Latarjet's nerve, adequate motility of the antropyloric pump is maintained while precluding pyloric spasm. Moreover, this ensures normal physiological emptying of the stomach and obviates the need for associated drainage procedures (Fig. 1). Experimentally, Daniel and Sarna have shown that preservation of the antropyloric branches of Latarjet's nerve in the dog [2] ensures adequate gastric emptying through vagovagal arcs.

In conventional surgery, this procedure had been well assessed by a large multicenter study on 605 patients with very good results, a low recurrence rate estimated at 1.5 % on 481 patients at 5 years [18]. Moreover, several control studies comparing the Taylor's procedure to highly selective vagotomy or truncal vagotomy concluded that posterior vagotomy and anterior seromyotomy is

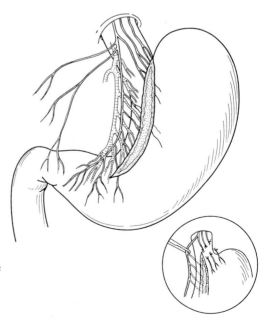

**Fig. 1.** Principle of the operation: the seromyotomy is led from the gastro-esophageal junction to the crus foot respecting the two inferior branches. *Inset*, Taylor's initial technique

as safe and efficient as other techniques but is more rapid than highly selective vagotomy, with the same advantages of gastric emptying and as efficient as truncal vagotomy. We therefore adopted this procedure in open surgery with the same experience as the authors [7] and with the same immediate results [6, 8].

In the emergency setting of perforated ulcer, peritonitis must be evaluated and treated first by irrigation and aspiration, the perforation then being closed. In the two procedures fibrin sealing is applied to secure the sutures of the sero-myotomy and of the perforated ulcer [9, 13, 14].

## Patient Selection

Preoperative evaluation of patients with chronic duodenal ulcer disease scheduled to undergo laparoscopic surgery is comparable to that in open surgery. Elective surgical correction of duodenal ulcer disease is indicated in patients in whom the diathesis is resistant to medical treatment in spite of perfect compliance to medical advice for at least 2 years, followed clinically and endoscopically with regular and well-conducted endoscopic and clinical control examinations and without intercurrent complications. Surgery is also recommended for patients who cannot comply with therapeutic advice correctly or cannot be followed regularly for geographic or socioeconomic reasons. As in elective open surgery, preoperative work-up includes evaluation of risk factors and the ulcer disease, which implies endoscopic and secretive investigations. Endoscopy demonstrates the ulcer which is usually linear without associated stenosis or hemorrhagic signs. Secretory tests include complete acidity evaluation with measurement of unstimulated acidity, basal acid output (BAO), and peak acid output (PAO) after stimulation with pentagastrin. Most patients refractory to medical treatment show marked hyperacidity. These tests are also useful in demonstrating postoperative reduction in acid output.

In the emergency setting video-laparoscopic intervention is indicated for patients seen within 12 h of perforation of their duodenal ulcer (chemical peritonitis). At this stage definitive treatment of the ulcer disease by Taylor's operation should be associated whenever feasible. If the patient is seen later than 12 h after perforation, management should be restricted to simple closure of the duodenal perforation.

## Surgical Procedure

As in traditional open surgery, general anesthesia and endotracheal intubation are used. The creation and continuation of pneumoperitoneum, the techniques of aspiration-lavage, thermocautery, and laser are the same as for other forms of laparoscopic surgery. We mention here only the problems specific to laparoscopic vagotomy, and which concern the positioning of the patient, instrumentation, approaches, exploration, and hemostatic techniques.

**Patient Positioning.**The patient is positioned in much the same way as for open cholecystectomy: the trunk is elevated 15°, lateral (left or right), tilting (also 15°) of the patient should be possible; a pillow roll or a bolster (10 cm) should be available. The patient is placed in the supine position, legs spread apart as in a two-team approach. The operating surgeon stands between the legs of the patient, the room nurse and first assistant are on the left and the second assistant on the right. The video-endoscopic system with irrigation/suction is placed on the left, and a second monitor with the laser unit is placed on the right. Electrocautery (Valleylab) and YAG laser systems (Microcontrol) complete the operating room units. The patient is prepared and draped, and the instruments are laid out as in traditional gastric surgery because an open operation may be required whenever laparoscopic surgery is deemed impossible or hazardous.

**Instrumentation.** In addition to the instruments usually utilized for this type of surgery, we recommend the following: (a) an angulated hook coagulator/dissector with a canal for evacuation of smoke (Karl Storz), (b) clip forceps (simple, Ligaclip; or multiple, Endoclip), (c) two Semm needle holders (Karl Storz), (d) 4/0 sutures with 2-cm curved or ski needles (Davis-Geck, Ethicon, U.S. Surgical), and (e) application systems for laser coagulation and collagen sealing (Karl Storz).

**Surgical Approaches.** Once the pneumoperitoneum has been created, the first trocar to be inserted is the video-laparoscopic 11-mm port introduced at one-third of the distance between the umbilicus and the xiphoid process (pl). Three further 5-mm and one 11-mm trocar are then inserted under visual control as shown in Fig. 2. These approaches are closed at the end of the operation by running intradermic sutures after complete desufflation of the abdomen and infiltration of the skin margins with local anesthesia in an effort to reduce postoperative pain.

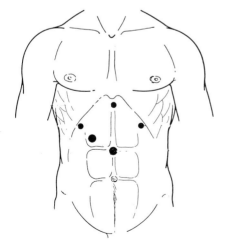

**Fig. 2.** Trocar insertion for video-laparoscope, palpator, graspers, and surgical instruments

**Exploration.** The abdominal cavity is explored as soon as the video-laparoscope is inserted. The surgeon should be sure that the operation is feasible without any major problems, and particularly that the liver can be retracted so that the operative area is visible. Associated lesions amenable to laparoscopic surgery are noted (adhesions, appendicitis, cholecystitis, biliary cyst). If the operation is impossible or seems dangerous or difficult, open surgery is of course preferred. The patient should be informed of this possibility beforehand.

**Hemostasis Procedures.** Several procedures are available: (a) The hook coagulator is used with monopolar current to coagulate small-caliber vessels safely. (b) The Nd-YAG laser coagulates superficial surfaces by contact fiber. (c) Titanium clips are used for the short gastric, left gastric, and small hepatic vessels which must be skeletonized first. (d) Suture ligation ensures hemostasis as in open surgery. All types of knots (flat, double, Roeder) may be made intra- or extracorporeally. Running suture is employed for seromyotomy. (e) Fibrin is spread on top to complete the closure of seromyotomy or of perforated ulcer.

## Technique of Posterior Truncal Vagotomy and Anterior Seromyotomy

The procedure consists of three steps: approach to the hiatal area, posterior vagotomy and anterior vagotomy.

**Approach of the Hiatal Area.** The left lobe of the liver is retracted with the xiphoid probe. The lesser sac is entered through an opening in the pars flaccida held between two angulated graspers which present the areolar tissues to the hook coagulator/dissector. Dissection is continued until the fleshy portion of the right crus is reached. If a left gastric vein or an accessory left hepatic artery is encountered, they may be divided between two clips as necessary.

**Posterior Truncal Vagotomy.** The two major landmarks for posterior truncal vagotomy are the caudate lobe and the right crus which can be grasped by the right-side grasping forceps and held to the right while the coagulator/dissector hook opens the pre-esophageal peritoneum. The abdominal esophagus is retracted to the left, allowing visualization of the areolar tissue where the posterior vagus nerve, easily recognized by its white color, can then be identified. While gentle traction is exerted on the nerve, adhesions are divided after coagulation and the nerve is transected between two clips. A fragment of the nerve is retrieved for histological verification.

**Anterior Seromyotomy.** The anterior aspect of the stomach is spread out between two grasping forceps. Starting at the esophagogastric junction, the future line of incision is outlined by light electrocoagulation parallel to and situated 1.5 cm from the lesser curvature. The line stops 5–7 cm from the pylorus at the level of the pes anserinus. The two most distal branches of the nerve are left intact to be sure that the antropyloric innervation remains functional. Seromyotomy is then performed with the hook coagulator using monopolar current, making equal use of the coagulation and division set at average intensity. The hook incises successively the serosal layer, the oblique, and then the circular superficial muscular layers. The two borders are then grasped and gently spread apart mechanically, thus breaking the remaining deep circular fibers. Electrocautery completes the division whenever necessary. Once the last muscular fibers have been divided, the mucosa can easily be identified by its typical blue color as it "pops" out of the incision. Because of the magnification, the surgeon can easily verify that no holes have been made inadvertently. During the incision two or three short vessels may be encountered. They are divided, as described in Taylor's technique, after identification with the hook coagulator/dissector which lifts them off the seromuscular layer. The ends may be clipped or suture ligated. It is of utmost importance that the incision be anatomically accurate with perfect hemostasis. Upon completion seromyotomy appears as a 7- to 8-mm trench in the gastric wall. Air is then injected through the nasogastric tube to make sure that there are no leaks. The seromyotomy is closed by an overlapping running suture, knotted at both ends, and secured by clips. Fibrin collagen application completes hemostasis (Fig. 3). Abdominal closure is performed without drainage.

### Closure of Perforated Ulcer

The perforation, usually on the anterior aspect of the duodenal bulb and generally 0.5–1 cm in diameter, is easily identified by video-laparoscopy, especially when gastric fluid can be seen to leak through the hole. The entire abdominal cavity is surveyed, evaluating the degree and extension of peritonitis, and free fluid is retrieved for bacterial identification. After initial irrigation and aspiration, the perforation may be closed in two manners. Simple closure can be achieved by using a Semm needle holder (Karl Storz) with a ski needle attached to a 15-cm-long thread. Two or three sutures are placed by half-key

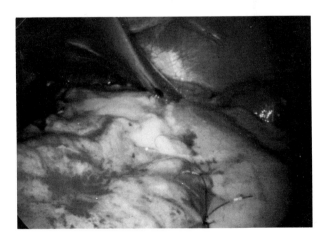

**Fig. 3.** Endoscopic pictures of the overlapping suture of the seromyotomy with fibrin sealant spread on its surface

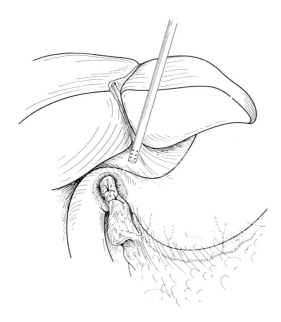

**Fig. 4.** Closure of the perforated ulcer by suture with omental patch

loops, attaching the omentum to each suture (Fig. 4). Fibrin sealant is then applied. Some authors use fibrin sealant only [13].

Hemostasis is checked, and final irrigation and aspiration complete the procedure. A nasogastric tube is positioned close to the suture. A drain is placed through the trocar in the right hypochondrium and is maintained under 30 mm H₂O negative pressure. The pneumoperitoneum is desufflated, and the abdominal wall is closed as in the vagotomy procedure described above.

### Postoperative Care

The nasogastric tube is left in place for 24 h after vagotomy and for 48 h after closure of perforation. The patient is discharged 3–5 days after vagotomy and 5–7 days after simple closure for perforation. Antibiotics are not used routinely for vagotomy but are given prophylactically for closure of perforation. As after cholecystectomy, postoperative pain is minimal and has practically disappeared since we have begun to inject a local anesthetic into the puncture holes. Whenever required, nonsteroid analgesics can be given.

### Present Experience

To date we have performed 90 operations for duodenal ulcer – 62 for chronic duodenal ulcer intractable to medical treatment and 28 for perforations. In elective cases results are comparable to those obtained in open techniques. There has been no operative complication, especially no injury of the mucosa and no conversion into open surgery even in the first cases. No death has occurred in this series and morbidity had been very low, consisting of one pneumothorax cured by drainage, one gastroesophageal reflux, two bezoars, and two mild cases of diarrhea. Immediate results have been very good, and the ulcers have disappeared after 1 month and acidity reduced by 8 % on follow-up acidity tests. At 2 years we have observed two recurrences compliant to medical treatment.

In an emergency case we have observed one death, in a patient aged 78 years, in the 24th h after the perforation. Laparoscopy showed the perforation to be located on the posterior wall, and the closure of perforation was judged not sufficient so that a conversion was performed. The patient died 3 days after in the intensive care unit of respiratory failure. Follow-up of the 27 other patients has been uneventful.

## Comments

Fibrin sealant has been utilized extensively in open surgery. Gelatine, cellulose, or collagen pads that are efficient in vitro have no adhesive power and are easily washed out by peritoneal liquid when used alone. The first biological glues based on gelatine, resorcine, formol, or cyanoacrylates proved to be difficult to use and histotoxic.

Although expensive and requiring external preparation, fibrin sealant has many advantages: easy manipulation, efficiency due to activation of the intrinsic coagulation, rapid drying, absence of tissular reaction in contact with antigenic stimulation, and quick resorption. Fibrin sealant also has an effect on enhancement of wound healing. Tissucol is more efficacious than other fibrin glues in digestive surgery. Indeed, the majority of surgical teams use Tissucol in open surgery to improve hemostasis. In laparoscopic surgery, fibrin sealant is of great use and must be applied without pulverization as this effect could increase the intra-abdominal $CO_2$ pressure leading to a risk of $CO_2$ embolism. In the laparoscopic treatment of duodenal ulcer by truncal vagotomy and anterior seromyotomy we originally applied fibrin sealant alone on the seromyotomy without any closure, and this proved to work very well. The experience of authors such as Mouret from Lyon in the repair of duodenal perforations by ulcer has proved that the use of fibrin sealant alone without any suture is also of great help in preventing postoperative leakage. Therefore we advocate the use of Tissucol on the seromyotomy after closure of this incision by sutures. The effect is to reduce the adhesion of the suture line and also to prevent blood loss and therefore diminishing the risk of infection and any other complications. We also currently use fibrin sealant on perforated duodenal ulcer after performing two sutures for an omental flap. This has proven efficacious in more than 30 patients [3, 4].

## Conclusion

Laparoscopic surgical treatment of duodenal ulcer disease is as safe and efficient as in open surgery. In elective cases, posterior truncal vagotomy and seromyotomy according the Taylor's procedure is full of promise and can be proposed for the patients resistant to medical treatment or noncompliant to maintenance drugs. Nevertheless, this new laparoscopic technique needs to be evaluated by multicenter control trial to evaluate not only the results of laparoscopic surgery but to compare them with medical treatment as to their efficacy and their cost effectiveness. In emergency cases, the laparoscopic approach is a very good solution for perforated ulcer as it allows a complete peritoneal toilet and closure of the perforation with minimal access surgery. In the two procedures, elective and emergency, fibrin sealant used in all cases secures the suture and approximation of tissues.

## References

1. Burge HW, Hutchinson JSF, Longland CJ, McLennan I, Mien DC, Rudick J, Tomkin AMB (1964) Selective nerve section in the prevention of post-vagotomy diarrhea. Lancet 1: 577
2. Daniel EE, Sarna SK (1986) Distribution of excitatory vagal fibres in canine gastric wall to central motility. Gastroenterology XX: 295–420
3. Frileux P, Boutelier P, Parc R, Peix JL, Thiebaut JB (1991) Evaluation de l'efficacité d'une nouvelle génération de compresses hémostatiques de collagène. Ann Chir 45: 126–133
4. Gouillat C, Tete B, Frering V, Saguier G, Ain JF, Bérard P (1990) Evaluation de l'efficacité de 2 colles de fibrine en chirurgie digestive: étude expérimentale chez le porc. Lyon Chir 86: 481–485
5. Hill GL, Barker MCJ (1978) Anterior highly selective vagotomy with posterior truncal vagotomy: a simple technique for denervating the parietal cell mass. Br J Surg 65: 702–705
6. Katkhouda N, Mouiel J (1991) A new surgical technique of treatment of chronic duodenal ulcer without laparotomy by videocoelioscopy. Am J Surg 161: 361–364
7. Mouiel J (1989) Actualités Digestives Médico-chirurgicales, 10th edn Masson, Paris, pp 20–22
8. Mouiel J, Katkhouda N, Gugenheim J, Fabiani P, Goubaux B (1990) Traitement de l'ulcère duodénal par vagotomie tronculaire postérieure et séromyotomie antérieure sous vidéo-laparoscopie. Note préliminaire avec présentation de film. Acad Chir (Paris) 116: 546–551
9. Mouiel J, Katkhouda N (1991) Laparoscopic truncal and selective vagotomy. In: Zucker K, Bailey RW (eds) Surgical laparoscopy. QMP, St Louis, pp 263–279
10. Mouiel J, Katkhouda N (1991) Traitement de l'ulcère duodénal non compliqué. In: Testas P, Delaitre B, Dubois F, De Watteville JC, Mouret PH, Perissat J, Samii K (eds) La chirurgie digestive par voie coelioscopique. Vigot, Paris, pp 137–145
11. Mouiel J, Katkhouda N (1991) Laparoscopic vagotomy in the treatment of chronic duodenal ulcer disease. In: Nyhus L, Berci G (eds) Problems in general surgery, vol 8.3, Lippincott, Philadelphia, pp 358–365
12. Mouiel J, Katkhouda N (1992) Laparoscopic anterior seromyotomy and posterior truncal vagotomy. In: Cuschieri A, Buess G, Perissat J (eds) Operative manual of endoscopic surgery. Springer, Berlin Heidelberg New York, pp 263–272
13. Mouret P, François Y, Vignal J, Barth X, Lombard-Platet R (1990) Laparoscopic treatment of perforated peptic ulcer. Br J Surg 77: 1006

14. Nathanson LK, Easter DW, Cuschieri A (1990) Laparoscopic repair/peritoneal toilet of perforated duodenal ulcer. Surg Endosc 4: 232–233
15. Smith GK, Farris JM (1963) Some observations upon selective gastric vagotomy. Arch Surg 86: 716
16. Taylor TV (1979) Lesser curve superficial seromyotomy. An operation for chronic duodenal ulcer. Br J Surg 66: 733-737
17. Taylor TV, MacLeod DAD, Gunn AA, MacLennan I (1982) Anterior lesser curve seromyotomy and posterior truncal vagotomy in the treatment of chronic duodenal ulcer. Lancet ii: 846–848
18. Taylor TV, Gunn AA, MacLoed DAD et al (1985) Morbidity and mortality after anterior lesser curve seromyotomy and posterior truncal vagotomy for duodenal ulcer. Br J Surg 72: 950–951

# Fibrin Sealing of the Liver Bed After Laparoscopic Cholecystectomy: A Prospective Randomized Study

P. Schrenk, R. Woisetschläger, and W. Wayand

## Abstract

The effect of fibrin sealing of the liver bed on the amount of postoperative drainage fluids after laparoscopic cholecystectomy was investigated prospectively in 20 patients (group I) and compared to 20 patients in whom hemostasis was achieved by electrocautery alone (group II). Mean drainage of fluids measured after 24 and 48 h postoperatively revealed a slight increase in group II patients (day 1, 26.6 ± 18.6 versus 36.5 ± 32.2 ml; day 2, 0 versus 2.3 ± 38.1 ml) but not of statistical significance. After uncomplicated laparoscopic cholecystectomy control of bleeding can be adequately achieved by electrocautery. However, in case of extensive and diffuse bleeding or aberrant bile duct fibrin sealing may be of advantage.

## Introduction

Sewing of the serosa of the liver bed after open cholecystectomy is performed routinely by some surgeons to achieve safe hemostasis of the gallbladder fossa and to provide adhesion prophylaxis [3]. While laparoscopic sewing of the liver bed is possible, it may be difficult and time consuming. Therefore sealing of the liver bed with fibrin glue (FG) seems to be a reliable and feasible alternative. The objective of the study was to investigate whether liver bed sealing with FG following laparoscopic cholecystectomy (LCHE) may be of advantage with regard to hemostasis compared to coagulation with electrocautery alone.

## Patients and Methods

Forty patients who underwent LCHE for symptomatic gallstones were randomly allocated to one of two groups. Those in group I received LCHE and FG sealing of the liver bed. After dissection of the gallbladder [5] and control of major liver bed bleedings the gallbladder fossa was sealed with 2 ml FG (Tissucol fibrin glue, 500 IU thrombin per 1 ml; Immuno, Vienna, Austria) applied through a 5-mm trocar in the right upper abdomen (Fig. 1). Those in group II

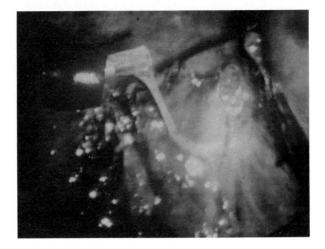

**Fig. 1.** Intraoperative photograph showing fibrin glue application through a 5-mm trocar in the upper right abdomen after laparoscopic dissection of the gallbladder

received LCHE without FG application. In group II patients bleedings due to dissection were controlled by use of electrocautery.

The two groups of patients were comparable with respect to age (I, 22–74 years, 44.7 ± 12.5; II, 26–75 years, 43.7 ± 14.5) and sex (I, male/female ratio 4/16; II, 4/16). The duration of surgery was slightly higher in group I patients (I, 30–90 min, 53.9 ± 15.0; II, 20–120 min, 60.7 ± 29.3) due to FG sealing. No patients with portal hypertension, coagulation disorders, or in whom the liver bed had to be rinsed postoperatively were included in the study.

Postoperatively a drain was placed beneath the liver bed, and drainage fluids were measured 24 and 48 h after surgery. Drains were removed 48 h postoperatively. Ultrasonography was performed on the second postoperative day to verify the amount of fluid collection in the liver bed.

Student's $t$-test was used for statistical analysis with $p < 0.05$ being taken as statistically significant.

### Results

The postoperative course was uncomplicated in both groups of patients. As seen in Table 1, mean drainage fluids measured 24 and 48 h postoperatively revealed a slightly increased volume in group II patients but without statistical significance. Ultrasonographic evaluation of the liver bed found normal results and revealed no major fluid collection due to intra- or postoperative bleeding.

### Discussion

Control of bleeding from the gallbladder fossa of the liver during laparoscopic cholecystectomy is usually achieved by the use of electrocautery [1, 5]. However, ultrasonographic evaluation of the liver bed has revealed tiny fluid collection in several cases, indicating insufficient intraoperative hemostasis in

**Table 1.** Mean drainage fluids (ml) 24 and 48 h after LCHE with (group I) or without (group II) FG sealing of the liver bed

|  | Group I (LCHE+FG) (*n* = 20) | Group II (LCHE−FG) (*n* = 20) |
|---|---|---|
| Drainage fluids after 24 h | 26.6+18.6 (0–50) | 36.5+32.2* (0–98) |
| Drainage fluids after 48 h | 0 | 2.3+38.1 (5–30) |
| Total drainage fluids | 20.6+18.6 (0–50) | 38.8+36.1* (0–110) |

* no significance between group I and II.

these patients [4]. FG has been applied to control liver hemorrhage in many instances and has provided effective hemostasis [2]. Therefore FG sealing may prevent or minimize postoperative fluid collection due to bleeding of the liver bed.

In this study FG sealing of the liver bed after LCHE was not associated with decreased postoperative drainage fluids. The amount of postoperative drainage fluids was comparable between the two groups regardless of whether the liver bed was sealed with FG or not. Additionally, ultrasonography of the liver bed revealed no differences in postoperative fluid deposits.

It may be concluded that in uncomplicated LCHE there is no need for FG sealing of the liver bed. Exact postoperative control of bleeding by electro-cautery should lead to similar results. However, in cases of extensive diffuse bleeding of the liver bed and aberrant bile ducts sealing with FG may be of advantage and seems to be a reliable and feasible alternative.

## *References*

1. Kent RB, Naughton MJ (1991) Hemostasis of the gallbladder fossa during laparoscopic cholecystectomy. Surg Laparosc Endosc 1: 104–105
2. Kram HB, Reuben BI, Fleming AW, Shoemaker WC (1988) Use of fibrin glue in hepatic trauma. J Trauma 28: 1195–1201
3. Kremer K, Lierse W, Platzer W, Schreiber HW, Weller S (eds) (1990) Chirurgische Operationslehre: Gallenblase, Gallenwege, Pancreas. Thieme, Stuttgart
4. Smith R, Kolyn D, Pymar H, Sauerbrei E, Pace RF (1992) Ultrasonographic and radiologic evaluation of patients after laparoscopic cholecystectomy. Can J Surg 35: 55–58
5. Woisetschläger R, Rieger R, Wayand W (1991) Die laparoskopische Cholecystektomie-Indikationsstellung, Technik und Ergebnisse. Osterr Therapiewoche 6 (12): 805–812

# Endoscopic Application of Fibrin Glue in the Treatment of Anastomotic Defects, Perforation, and Fistulas in the Gastrointestinal Tract

H. GROITL, T. HORBACH, R. STANGL, and J. SCHEELE

## Abstract

Since December 1984 we have applied fibrin glue endoscopically in the treatment of anastomotic defects, fistulas, and perforation in the upper and lower gastrointestinal tracts in a total of 84 patients. Our patient group consisted of 51 patients with intrathoracic complications after esophageal or stomach surgery and 33 patients with anastomotic defect after colorectal operations or in colorectal or rectovaginal fistulas. Using this approach perianastomotic abscess cavities could be cleansed quickly, and granulation tissue growth and complete healing were promoted in 44 of 51 patients with anastomotic defect in the upper gastrointestinal tract. In the lower gastrointestinal tract the outcome of treatment of anastomotic defects was also good, but not so for fistula treatment. Endoscopic application of fibrin glue is an effective and direct form of biological treatment which puts little strain on the patient.

## Introduction

Since the 1980s fibrin glue has found increasing use in many areas of surgery. With the development of double- and four-lumen catheters in 1984 the components of the glue* can be mixed just before application via the endoscope, and the glue can then be applied to the wound surface, sprayed on, or even injected [1–13].

## Materials and Methods

From 1 December 1985 to 30 November 1993 fibrin glue was applied endoscopically in the treatment of lesions in the upper gastrointestinal tract (GIT) in 51 consecutive patients and in the lower GIT in 33 patients.

**Upper Intestinal Tract.** The patient group treated with fibrin in the upper GIT consisted of 13 women and 38 men ranging in age from 17 to 79 years. Of these patients 43 presented with anastomotic defects after the following surgical

---

* Tissucol Duo S, human fibrinogen, human thrombin, steam treated

interventions: esophageal resection and esophagogastrostomy ($n = 18$), colonic interposition after esophageal resection ($n = 1$), gastrectomy and Roux-en-Y anastomosis ($n = 24$). In eight patients iatrogenic perforations, chronic fistulas, and esophageal lesions subsequent to myotomy had developed. In three cases leakage was detected at clinical examination and in a further 48 at endoscopic or radiological examinations. In ten patients, in five of whom Gastrografin passage had been normal, the defect could only be confirmed endoscopically. In eight patients previous operative treatment had been unsuccessful. Primary septic complications were present to a greater or lesser degree in all 51 patients, and 33 of them required intensive care. Organic functional disturbances developed which necessitated hemofiltration or mechanical ventilation in 22 patients.

**Lower Gastrointestinal Tract.** The patient group treated with fibrin in the lower GIT consisted of 33 patients, 14 women and 19 men, ranging in age from 24 to 84 years. Fibrin glue was used to treat anastomotic defects after colorectal surgery ($n = 14$) and due to colorectal ($n = 13$) or rectovaginal ($n = 6$) fistulas. Diagnosis was secured exclusively by endoscopy in 13 patients and by a combination of endoscopic and radiological methods in 20. Nine of the 14 patients with anastomotic defects required intensive care for septic complications, in particular peritonitis. In one patient treatment had been preceded by unsuccessful operative revision. The 19 fistula patients were in good general condition at the beginning of treatment.

**Technique.** In all patients the first treatment step involved thorough flushing with physiological saline to cleanse the abscess cavity or fistular canal, initially one to three times daily via the endoscope. Then fibrin was applied to the cleansed surface area of the wound. The amount and frequency of application depended on the nature of the wound and the patient's condition. Special attention was paid to good drainage of the abscess or fistula, usually open drainage without suction.

## Results

Treatment according to the method described above was successful in 44 patients of the group with wounds in the upper GIT (86%). In these individuals the abscess cavities were cleansed, granulation tissue had developed, and the wound had healed in a relatively short time. In 64% less than five fibrin applications were necessary to stabilize the individual patient clinically and, by promoting growth of granulation tissue, for the wound to close. The promising results of the first treatments prompted us in the further course of the study to treat lesions with a diameter of 10 cm and more, which required a greater number of applications and more fibrin. In nine patients the fistula had closed, but anastomotic stenosis developed which required dilatation or endoscopic cauterization. Seven patients died of septic complications already existing at the onset of treatment. In two patients complete healing could not be achieved despite intensive cleansing and fibrin application; the chronic fistulas had to be closed surgically after the clinical condition of these individuals had stabilized.

This regimen was successful in 20 patients (61 %) treated in the lower GIT; 11 of the 14 anastomotic defects (79 %) could be repaired permanently. However, in only five of 13 patients with colorectal fistulas (38 %) and four of six patients with rectovaginal fistulas was fibrin glue treatment completely effective, usually being less successful in patients with long-term, chronic fistulas and those who had chronic infections. The duration of treatment was considerably longer (up to 16 weeks) and more frequent in the lower GIT than in the upper GIT.

## Discussion

Further trauma to patients – as would occur, for example, at rethoracotomy or relaparotomy – can be avoided if fibrin is applied endoscopically, and endoscopy does fulfill all the requirements of antiseptic surgery as regards opening, cleansing, and drainage. In contrast to conventional surgery, during which healthy tissue is injured and frequently also contaminated, the neighboring structures are not affected during endoscopic procedures. The strain under which a patient often already weakened by septic complications is put can be kept to a minimum with short, low-stress endoscopic procedures. Patients who are not in stable condition do not have to be moved from the intensive care unit to another ward. Space (operating rooms) and personnel (endoscopists and assistants – in contrast to operating team, anesthetist, and intensive care staff) requirements are not problematic. After treatment in the hospital has been successfully initiated, therapy can often be continued on an outpatient basis.

Postoperative anastomotic defects can be successfully treated. In contrast, outcome of chronic wound treatment is relatively poor, in particular in the lower GIT. Along with very promising good individual outcomes one finds those patients with long-term, frustrating courses. Here the therapeutic approach must be considered on an individual basis, whereby fibrin treatment, which involves less strain on the patient, is generally preferable to surgery, since the outcome of surgery is equally unpredictable.

Summarizing our results we see three significant advantages of endoscopic fibrin application: (a) Drainage of mediastinal or pararectal abscesses associated with anastomotic defects is effective, and septic complications can often be avoided if treatment is begun early. (b) Fibrin glue aids in wound cleansing and promotes healing by stimulating the development of granulation tissue so that even extremely large wounds heal well. (c) Endoscopy is usually more reliable than, for example, radiological examination in identifying such lesions in the GIT, and treatment can be initiated immediately (Fig. 1).

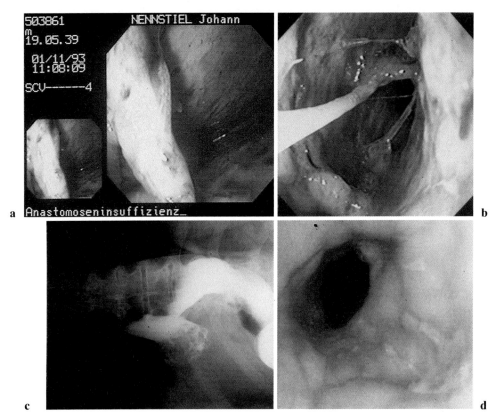

**Fig. 1a–d.** Esophageal resection and reconstruction using right abdominal thoracic approach in a 54-year-old man who had squamous cell carcinoma of the esophagus (pT1, pN0, UICC I, R 0). **a** Endoscopic view of the anastomosis on the seventh postoperative day. Defect of about 30 % of the circumference seen on the *right* in the mediastinum. **b** Clean granulation tissue in the perianastomotic cavity on the 22nd postoperative day after fibrin sealing. **c** There is still extensive leakage in the cavity on the 35th postoperative day. **d** Follow-up examination of the anastomosis 3½ months after release from the hospital. The patient had been released from the hospital on the 51st postoperative day and was eating normally at that time

## References

1. Despang F (1992) Endoskopischer Fistelverschluß postoperativer Anastomoseninsuffizienzen im Gastrointestinaltrakt durch Fibrinklebung. In: Gebhardt C (ed) Fibrinklebung in der Allgemein- und Unfallchirurgie, Orthopädie, Kinder- und Thoraxchirurgie. Springer, Berlin Heidelberg New York, pp 75–77
2. Eimiller A (1988) Behandlung von Fisteln bei M. Crohn durch Fibrinklebung. In: Manegold BC, Jung M (eds) Fibrinklebung in der Endoskopie. Springer, Berlin Heidelberg New York, pp 147–151
3. Groitl H, Scheele J (1987) Erste Erfahrung mit der endoskopischen Anwendung eines Fibrinklebers am oberen Gastrointestinaltrakt. Z Herz Thorax Gefasschir [Suppl] 1: 74–78

4. Groitl H, Scheele J (1987) First experiences with endoscopic application of fibrin tissue adhesive in the upper gastrointestinal tract. Surg Endosc 1: 93–97
5. Jung M (1988) Verklebung von Fisteln am Ösophagus. In: Manegold BC, Jung M (eds) Fibrinklebung in der Endoskopie. Springer, Berlin Heidelberg New York, pp 47–54
6. Jung M, Brands W, Manegold BC (1987) Endoskopische Fibrinklebung. Z Herz Thorax Gefasschir 1 [Suppl 1]: 79–83
7. Lange V (1988) Endoskopischer Verschluß gastrointestinaler Fisteln. In: Manegold BC, Jung M (eds) Fibrinklebung in der Endoskopie. Springer, Berlin Heidelberg New York, pp 125–160
8. Lange V, Meyer G (1990) Fistuloscopy – an adjuvant technique for sealing gastrointestinal fistulae. Surg Endosc 4: 212–216
9. Lange V, Meyer G, Rau H, Mewes A (1992) Endoskopische Intervention bei postoperativen Fisteln. In: Gebhardt C (ed) Fibrinklebung in der Allgemein- und Unfallchirurgie, Orthopädie, Kinder- und Thoraxchirurgie, Springer, Berlin Heidelberg New York, pp 99-106
10. Lange V, Meyer G, Rau H, Schildberg FW (1992) Endoskopische Therapie gastrointestinaler Fisteln. Chir Gastroenterol 8: 344–349
11. Papadopoulos I, Schnapka B, Kelami A (1987) Verschluß von Blasen-Scheiden-Fisteln im Experiment und in der Klinik mit Hilfe von Humanfibrinkleber. In: Kubli F, Schmidt W, Gauwerky J (eds) Fibrinklebung in der Frauenheilkunde und Geburtshilfe. Springer, Berlin Heidelberg New York, pp 146–151
12. Waclawiczek H-W, Heinermann M, Meiser G, Lexer G (1992) Verhütung bzw. Behandlung postoperativer Fisteln – neue Indikationen für die Fibrinklebung. Wien Klin Wochenschr 104: 474–481
13. Wenzel M (1985) Fistelverschluß mit Fibrinkleber. Chir Prax 34: 267–272
14. Widmaier G (1987) Anwendung von Fibrinkleber bei der Behandlung von Vesico-Vaginal-Fisteln. In: Kubli F, Schmidt W, Gauwerky J (eds) Fibrinklebung in der Frauenheilkunde und Geburtshilfe. Springer, Berlin Heidelberg New York, pp 152–153
15. Wolf N (1988) Indikationen zur Fibrinklebung in der Proktologie. In: Manegold BC, Jung M (eds) Fibrinklebung in der Endoskopie. Springer, Berlin Heidelberg New York, pp 161–163

# Fibrin Sealing in Laparoscopic Colorectal Surgery

T. RECK, C. SCHNEIDER, I. SCHNEIDER, I. GASTINGER, and F. KÖCKERLING

## Abstract

Successful laparoscopic colorectal surgery depends essentially on the following requirements: (a) a reliable anastomotic technique, (b) lymph node dissection according to the principles of oncological radicality and (c) the specimen removal technique. In extensive animal studies we have developed a laparoscopic operative method for deep rectal carcinoma by abdominoperineal rectum extirpation with high ligation of the inferior mesenteric artery. The first clinical use of the method was in January 1992. From January to October we successfully operated on ten patients using the new technique; no severe complications were observed. Although Well's transabdominal rectopexy to correct rectum prolapse is technically simple and yields good results, a minimally invasive procedure is desirable in the treatment of this benign condition. Therefore we developed a laparoscopic rectopexy technique based on Well's method in animal models. In principle, laparoscopic rectopexy does not differ greatly from the intra-abdominal approach used in Well's rectopexy, but the techniques applied in the individual steps must be adapted for laparoscopic application. We have successfully performed this operation without any complications in six patients with complete prolapse of the rectum. For the treatment of residual bleeding in the pelvic region and for additional fixation of the rectum to the sacrum in Well's procedure, fibrin sealing has been found very useful.

## Introduction

Working on laparoscopic colorectal surgery we were confronted with various problems which might be solved by laparoscopic fibrin sealing. First two well-proved colorectal surgical procedures at our institution, laparoscopic abdominoperineal rectum excision and laparoscopic rectopexy according to Well's method, are demonstrated, emphasizing the possible indications for fibrin sealing. These indications are then examined in an experimental animal study.

## Materials and Methods

### Operative Procedure for Laparoscopic Abdominoperineal Rectum Excision

The patient's position, arrangement of the equipment, and trocar incisions have been described previously [3]. First, mobilization of the mesocolon along the fascia of Gerota up to the aorta is performed by blunt dissection. After incision of the peritoneum the ureter is displayed at the crossing point of the common iliac artery. The further mobilization of the mesocolon from the fascia of Gerota is made only so far in the direction of the splenic flexure as it is necessary for a traction-free establishment of the colostomy.

Pushing the mesocolon with two swabs on a stick to the left, we divide the right peritoneum above the aorta followed by dissection down to the pelvic floor. For the dorsal mobilization of the rectum we push the mesorectum with two swabs on a stick into a ventral direction so that the retrorectal space is visualized by dissection. Scissor dissection of the presacral connective tissue is performed as far down to the pelvic floor as possible.

For a safe division of the mesentery and the larger vessels the linear stapler has shown good results. For this purpose the vessel trunk of the mesenteric artery is visualized in front of the aorta. The inferior mesenteric vessels, the mesentery of the descending colon passing into the sigmoid colon, and the colon itself are now divided step by step with the linear stapler via the trocars on the right or left side. In preparation for the following pelvic dissection, the distal colon end is caught with a forceps for traction into a cranioventral direction. The pelvic dissection requires a division of the ligaments close to the pelvic wall using electrocautery and endoclips.

After the anterior dissection of the rectum is performed in the recess of the fascia of Denonvilliers the rectum can be mobilized completely down to the levator ani muscle, remaining small residual bleedings must be controlled. Finally, the colostomy is established. For this purpose the 12-mm trocar is replaced by a 20-mm trocar. The fascia and skin are incised, and the colon stump is grasped with a forceps and withdrawn together with the 20-mm trocar. After finishing the sacral phase of the operation the lesser pelvis is checked again. Occasionally some problems arise from diffuse bleeding in this phase, and a very careful and proper hemostatis must be achieved.

### Operative Procedure for Laparoscopic Rectopexy

Although Well's transabdominal rectopexy to correct rectum prolapse is technically simple and yields good results, a minimally invasive procedure is desirable in the treatment of this benign condition. We therefore developed a laparoscopic rectopexy technique in animal models and have successfully used it in six patients [1].

The dorsal and lateral mobilization of the rectum is comparable to that by the laparoscopic abdominoperineal rectum excision described above. After the marlex mesh is taken into the abdominal cavity and rolled out on the fascia of

Waldeyer, it must be fixed by sutures. The problem is to avoid any injury of the presacral vessels.

The mobilized rectum is caught with two swabs on a stick for traction into a cranial direction. The marlex mesh must be carefully fixed again with seromuscular sutures exactly without contaminating the prosthetic material by colonic bacteria.

## Animal Study

In an experimental study we attempted to examine the following possible indications for fibrin sealing derived from our clinical experience in patient cases:

- Diffuse bleeding in the lesser pelvis after rectum excision
- Fixation of the marlex mesh to the fascia of Waldeyer for rectopexy
- Fixation of the mobilized rectum to the marlex mesh
- Fibrin sealing to cover the whole marlex mesh after rectopexy to avoid postoperative complicated adhesions with the small bowel
- Fibrin sealing of laparoscopic colon anastomosis as described previously [2]

In our experiment we used minipigs with an average weight of 20 kg ($n = 5$). Feed was withdrawn 2 days before; water was given ad libitum for colonic lavage. After anesthesia was induced with 0.3 g hexobarbital and 30–40 mg suxamethonium intravenously, the trachea was intubated. Anesthesia was maintained by ventilation with a nitrous oxide/oxygen (70 %/30 %) mixture using a respirator and droperidol/fentanyl intravenously as a continuous infusion. Pancuronium was given for long-term relaxation. Heart rate and blood pressure were monitored continuously, blood gas and acidbase content every 30 minutes. Fibrin glue was used as spray application with the Tissomat together with a specially designed three-luminal catheter for a laparoscopic procedure. Furthermore, conventional flexible application catheters, known from endoscopy, and rigid two-luminal metal catheters were examined, all of them adaptable to a 5-mm trocar.

## Results

### Clinical Study

Since January 1992 ten patients with a carcinoma of the lower rectum have undergone the above laparoscopic operation. There were no postoperative complications, with the exception of two patients with retarded healing process of the perineal wound. The operating procedure lasted between 4,5 and 6 h. Two patients underwent palliative excision of the rectum with existing pulmonary and hepatic metastases. After laparoscopic abdominoperineal excision of the rectum the postoperative course was more favorable both for the patients and for the nursing staff. The patients hardly complained of abdominal pain but merely of a painful perineal wound. As a rule the colostomy discharged already on the 2nd or 3rd postoperative day; oral feeding can be recommended earlier.

Since April 1992 six patients with a rectum prolapse have received laparoscopic rectopexy using Well's method. There were no intraoperative or postoperative complications. All patients benefited from this minimally invasive procedure. Although long-term results are not yet available, the danger of recurrence should be low because laparoscopic rectopexy does not differ greatly in principle from the intra-abdominal approach used in Well's rectopexy. Only the techniques used in the individual steps were adapted for a laparoscopic method.

*Animal Study*

In our hands the spray application of fibrin glue was not appropriate to the pneumoperitoneum within the closed abdominal cavity because the fibrin mist soon covered the optic lens and reduced the overview. Furthermore, we could not apply enough fibrin glue to control local bleeding in the lower pelvis. In contrast, using a conventional method applying 1 ml fibrin glue with a double-luminal flexible catheter hemostasis could be achieved easily (Fig. 1).

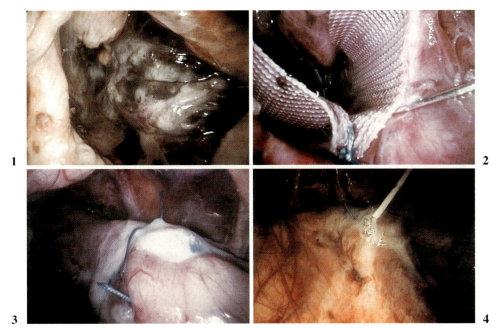

**Fig. 1** Application of fibrin glue to the lower pelvic cavity after rectum excision

**Fig. 2** Fixation of the marlex mesh to the fascia of Waldeyer for rectopexy (application with a rigid metal catheter)

**Fig. 3** Fibrin sealing of the marlex mesh and the mobilized rectum

**Fig. 4** Fibrin sealing of laparoscopic colon anastomosis

In the experimental study for laparoscopic rectopexy we fixed the marlex mesh only with two temporary sutures to the fascia of Waldeyer. Then we performed fibrin sealing. For this purpose the fibrin glue was syringed behind the mesh using the rigid metal catheter designed for laparoscopic application. We were thus able to reduce the risk of injuring presacral vessels by avoiding further sutures (Fig. 2).

Fibrin sealing for the fixation of the mobilized rectum to the marlex mesh avoids many colonic sutures with the risk of bacterial contamination of the prosthetic material. With 2 ml fibrin glue we could cover the whole marlex mesh and secured the sealing of the prosthetic implant which might reduce early adhesions to the small bowel (Fig. 3).

Finally, there was no problem applying fibrin glue to laparoscopic colon anastomoses carried out with the triple-stapling technique to obtain sealing of the intestinal anastomosis [2] (Fig. 4).

## *Discussion*

Particularly in laparoscopic colorectal surgery we are confronted with technical problems which could comfortably be solved by an open procedure as laparotomy. Nevertheless the application of fibrin sealing makes some individual steps in laparoscopic technique less troublesome. Furthermore, it probably reduces the time of operation. Diffuse bleeding in the lesser pelvis after rectum excision is sometimes a problem even in open surgery by laparotomy. The available laparoscopic instruments increase the problem because the means for achieving hemostasis are more difficult. In these situations fibrin glue can be recommended and provides good results.

The spray applicator using pressurized gas with the Tissomat did not prove satisfying in our hands because the optic lens became polluted by the fibrin glue mist, although temporary opening the trocar valve the risk of a gas embolism by increasing the intra-abdominal pressure cannot be ruled out. Further studies are necessary before a laparoscopic spray application can be used safely. Even the manufacturers (Immuno, Heidelberg) warn of any application of pressurized gas within a closed cavity. It might be associated with a potential risk of gas emphysema, tissue rupture, and air embolism [5].

The simplest means for fibrin application during laparoscopy is to take the conventional disposable catheter sets for endoscopy which are long enough for the purposes mentioned above. Taking the end of the catheter with a laparoscopic forceps, each point of the abdominal cavity can be reached easily for depositing of fibrin glue.

Laparoscopic rectopexy with a marlex mesh may be a good indication for fibrin sealing, as demonstrated above. Nevertheless long-term studies will show whether it works reliably.

Whether laparoscopic colon anastomosis should be sealed by fibrin glue cannot be decided because of our still limited experience. According to Waclawiczek [4], there is in principle no indication for a strengthening of a colon anastomosis by fibrin sealing. Perhaps using the new laparoscopic triple-stapling technique [2], there may be benefit in reducing the rate of anastomotic leakage.

## References

1. Köckerling F, Gastinger I, Gall CW, Schneider B, Krause W, Gall FP (1992) Laparoskopische Rectopexie. Minimal Invasive Chir 1: 68–72
2. Köckerling F, Gastinger I, Schneider B, Krause W, Gall FP (1992) Laparoskopische kolorektale Chirurgie: Kolon- und Rektumanastomosen in Triple-Stapling-Technique. Minimal Invasive Chir 1: 44–50
3. Köckerling F, Gastinger I, Schneider B, Krause W, Gall FP (1992) Laparoskopische abdominoperineale Rektumexstirpation mit hoher Durchtrennung der Arteria mesenterica inferior. Chirurg 63: 345–348
4. Waclawiczek HW, Boeckl O (1992) Ist die Anastomosensicherung mit Fibrinkleber am Gastrointestinaltrakt noch indiziert? In: Gebhardt C (ed) Fibrinklebung in der Allgemein- und Unfallchirurgie, Orthopädie, Kinder- und Thoraxchirurgie. Springer, Berlin Heidelberg New York, p 78–86
5. Wirth C, Odar J (1992) Applikationstechniken bei der Fibrinklebung. In: Gebhardt C (ed) Fibrinklebung in der Allgemein- und Unfallchirurgie, Orthopädie, Kinder- und Thoraxchirurgie. Springer, Berlin Heidelberg New York, p 17–25

# The Use of Fibrin Glue in Sclerotherapy for Esophageal Varices: Preliminary Results of a Controlled Prospective Study

F. RUCKTÄSCHEL, K. ZIEGLER, and T. ZIMMER

## Abstract

In a randomized prospective study 26 patients with esophageal varices were treated after a first bleeding episode with either fibrin or polidocanol, both strictly injected intravariceal. Treatments were repeated until obliteration of varices, based on endoscopic and endosonographic evaluation, was achieved. Fourteen patients were treated with polidocanol and 12 with fibrin. There were no significant differences in stage of liver disease between the two groups. Complete variceal obliteration was achieved in six patients treated with polidocanol (42.8 %) and nine patients in the fibrin group (75 %). An average of 4 treatments with polidocanol and 5.2 treatments with fibrin was necessary. During therapy with polidocanol 11 episodes of rebleeding occurred in six patients. In the fibrin group only one patient suffered from two episodes of rebleeding. Esophageal ulcers caused by sclerotherapy were observed in 56.1 % of polidocanol treatments and 8.7 % of fibrin treatments. In neither group were changes of laboratory values or thrombembolic complications observed. These preliminary results show that it is possible to achieve a higher rate of obliteration with fewer complications using fibrin than with polidocanol. Therefore, we propose treating acute esophageal variceal bleeding with fibrin, especially in all patients with a higher risk of complications.

## Introduction

The disease of liver cirrhosis is associated with high morbidity and mortality [10]. Acute bleeding of esophageal varices is the most frequent cause of death after liver failure [2, 5, 12, 20]. According to present data, the lethality of the first bleeding episode is about 30 %–40 % [5, 15]. In those surviving the first incident the risk of rebleeding is about 70 % [1, 11]. Therefore, there are two indications for the therapeutic approach: treatment for acute bleeding and prevention of rebleeding episodes.

There are various therapeutic procedures for treating acute esophageal variceal bleeding: Thermic procedures (laser coagulation) [10], mechanical blood staunching (Sengstaken-Blakermore tube) [12, 18], surgical therapy (shunt/emergency shunt operation) [2, 3], and injection therapy (endoscopic sclerotherapy) [5, 16]. Thermic procedures and mechanical blood staunching are able to stop bleeding only temporarily. Because of the high mortality (23 %–52 %) under shunt therapy [7] and the potential deterioration of liver function due to pathophysical mechanism [2, 3] injection sclerotherapy has proved to be the first choice in acute esophageal variceal bleeding and the prophylaxis of rebleeding episodes. Since its first description in the year 1939 [4] endoscopic sclerotherapy has been successful in numerous trials for the treatment of acute esophageal variceal bleeding [9] and for long-term prophylactic treatment [8, 19]. With this treatment the intra- and/or paravasal application of a drug induces an obliteration of varicose veins due to tissue scaring [20]. However, the common drugs taken for endoscopic sclerotherapy still cause considerable adverse effects [16]. The application of sclerosants such as polidocanol, ethanolaminoleate, and histoacryl is often associated with mucosal damage of the esophagus, including severe transmural ulceration. Some 60 %–80 % of such ulcers appear after sclerotherapy with polidocanol injection [12].

Rebleeding from these lesions is a serious problem especially for patients with poor liver function of patients with contraindications for other therapeutic procedures such as portocaval shunt operation. For this reason it is necessary to search for new, toxic sclerosants.

Today with a two-compound tissue glue based on fibrin there is a nontoxic drug able to stop bleeding from gastrointestinal ulcers by endoscopic injection. It may also prove capable of inducing variceal obliteration by clot formation after intravariceal injection. We therefore compared in a controlled, randomized study the effectiveness of polidocanol, the most established sclerosant, versus fibrin in sclerotherapy for acute esophageal variceal bleeding.

## Patients and Methods

For this trial Tissucol was used, a fibrin sealant in the form of a two-compound application set, manufactured by Immuno (Heidelberg). Its production is based on the use of fresh human plasma. For this product there has only been used hepatitis B surface antigen negative, GPT-controlled specimens. The donor material was checked for HIV and since July 1992 for hepatitis C virus. In several studies a risk for the transfer of hepatitis or immunodeficiency viruses has in all probability been excluded [6, 13, 14, 17].

To date, 26 patients have entered the program (14 men, 12 women; average age 60.9 years). They were randomized after a first bleeding episode from esophageal varices according to their stage of liver disease. The stage of liver disease was determined using Child's classification. In stages A, B, and C there were 5, 5, and 2 patients, respectively, in the fibrin sealant group and 6, 6, and 2 in the polidocanol group.

Sclerotherapy followed according to the randomization list either with fibrin sealant or with polidocanol. In acute bleeding primary blood staunching was achieved by the Sengstaken-Blakemore tube.

Injection sclerotherapy was carried out in the bleeding-free interval using a flexible balloon scleroscope (Olympus). Patients were first premedicated by the injection of 2–5 mg midazolam (Dormicum), 2–5 mg Triflupromazine (Psyquil), and 5–15 mg pentazocine (Fortral). Under proximal blockade for the prevention of intravariceal flowing the strictly intravariceal injection of the sclerosant was undertaken through a flexible needle. Depending on the patients' allocation in the randomization list each vessel was treated either with 4–8 ml polidocanol or 2–3 ml fibrin sealant. The injection of polidocanol as one-compound drug was as a bolus in each vessel. In contrast, we applied the fibrin sealant in sequent-technique. In this way the components were kept apart inside the needle through interposed injection of aq. dest. to avoid intraluminal clotting of the two components. According to first trials with single- and double-luminal needles the sequential injection with monoluminal needles has been the most advantageous.

Initial filling of the needle with aq. dest. was followed by: 1 ml fibrinogen compound, 1 ml aq. dest., 1 ml thrombin compound, and 1 ml aq. dest. Consequently, the above scheme was repeated three times for the application of 3 ml fibrin sealant. Four to six days after sclerotherapy endoscopic and endosonographic evaluation was performed. Vessels still open were treated again. Endoscopic findings were the standard for this. In cases of ulcerations findings were controlled 3 weeks later in regard to healing and variceal obliteration. The treatments were repeated until full obliteration of all varices was achieved. When this goal was reached, endoscopic and endosonographic evaluation was repeated after 3 weeks. If full obliteration remained, the patients entered a cycle of 3-month-controls (Fig. 1).

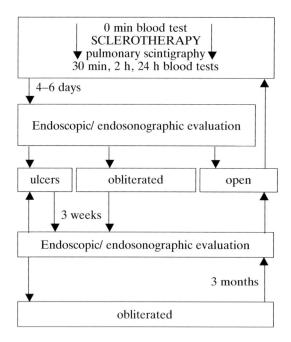

**Fig. 1** Treatment scheme

Postoperative observation included the registration of breathing, pulse, blood pressure, and body temperature. Blood tests before and after sclerotherapy (30 min, 2 h, 24 h) determined: partial thromboplastin time, fibrinogen, fibrin split product, thrombin-antithrombin complex, partial thromboplastin time, thromboplastin time, d-dimers, and blood count including thrombocytes. Pulmonary embolism due to therapy was excluded through pulmonary scintigraphy. Further explorations were undertaken in cases of undesirable symptoms.

## Results

Complete variceal obliteration has been achieved in 9 of 12 patients (75 %) treated with fibrin sealant. In the polidocanol group 6 of 14 patients were treated successfully (42 %). An average of 4 treatments with polidocanol and 5.2 treatments with fibrin sealant were necessary (Table 1).

Under therapy with polidocanol 11 episodes of rebleeding occurred in 6/14 patients. A four of those died during bleeding, leading to a rebleeding rate of 42.6 %. Eight of these bleedings were treated with Sengstaken-Blakemore tube; 60 blood transfusions were undertaken, and two patients were respirated under intubation. During therapy with fibrin sealant only one patient suffered from two episodes of rebleeding, leading to a rebleeding rate of 8.3 %. Except for the application of seven blood transfusions, no further therapeutic measures were necessary.

Esophageal ulcers were observed after 23 of 41 polidocanol sessions (56.1 %). Partially, these ulcers persisted for a long time and caused undesirable extensions of therapy. Six of 69 fibrin sessions (8.7 %) caused esophageal ulcerations. In general, healing was completed in between 3 weeks.

Five of 14 patients died under therapy with polidocanol, one due to renal failure and four during rebleeding episodes. During therapy with fibrin sealant 1/12 patients died due to liver failure.

The laboratory parameters showed no significant differences between the study groups. There were no pathological changes in clotting tests. There was no pulmonary embolism in any of the study groups. This was demonstrated by clinical observation and corroborated by pulmonary scintigraphy. There were no clinical signs of allergic reactions, either under therapy with polidocanol or under that with fibrin-sealant.

**Table 1.** Variceal obliteration

| Child group | Fibrin sealant | | Polidocanol | |
|---|---|---|---|---|
| | $n$ | % | $n$ | % |
| A | 4/5 | 80 | 3/6 | 50 |
| B | 4/5 | 80 | 3/6 | 50 |
| C | 1/2 | 50 | 0/2 | 0 |
| Total | 9/12 | 75 | 6/14 | 42 |

## Discussion

As the rates of occlusion show, fibrin sealant is able to induce esophageal variceal obliteration. The percentage of successful cases is higher than with polidocanol. However, the average number of treatments necessary for complete obliteration is higher with fibrin sealant. The survival rate at 1-year follow-up is higher for patients treated with fibrin sealant. There were no systemic side effects from the fibrin sealant. There were fewer local complications such as ulcerations and erosions; thus, patients treated with fibrin sealant had a lower rebleeding rate than those treated with polidocanol.

On the one hand, it is more expensive to treat patients with fibrin sealant than with polidocanol. These costs are due to the higher price of the drug and to the increased number of treatments necessary. On the other, fibrin sealant enables a cost decrease by avoiding rebleeding episodes as fewer transfusions and intensive care are needed. These preliminary results show that it is advantageous to use fibrin sealant in sclerotherapy of acute esophageal variceal bleeding especially for patients in bad clinical condition due to bleeding. A further indication is prophylactic sclerotherapy for high-risk patients with poor liver function, contraindication for shunt therapy, or with bleeding ulcers conditioned by sclerotherapy.

## References

1. Cales P, Pascal JP (1988) Histoire naturelle des varices oesophagiennes au cours de la cirrhose (de la naissance à la rupture). Gastroenterol Clin Biol. 12: 245.
2. Cello JP, Grendell JH, Crass RA (1984). Endoscopic sclerotherapy versus portocaval shunt in patients with severe cirrhosis and variceal hemorrhage. N Engl J Med 311 (25): 1589–1594.
3. Cello JP, Grendel JH, Crass RA (1987) Endoscopic sclerotherapy versus portocaval shunt in patients with severe cirrhosis and acute variceal hemorrhage. Long term follow-up. N Engl J Med 316 (1): 11–15
4. Crafoord C, Frenckner P (1939) New surgical treatment of varicose veins of the oesophagus. Acta Otolaryngol (Stockh) 27: 422–429
5. Denk H (1977) Die endoskopische Behandlung von Ösophagusvarizen. Chirurg 48: 212–218
6. Eder G, Neumann M, Cervenka R (1986) Preliminary results of a randomized controlled study on the risk of hepatitis transmission of a two-component fibrin-sealant (Tissucol/Tisseel) In: Schlag G (ed) Fibrin sealant in operative medicine. Springer, Berlin Heidelberg New York, pp 51–59
7. Häring R (1977) Chirurgische Notfallmaßnahmen bei der massiven Ösophagusvarizenblutung. Dtsch Med Wochenschr 102: 289–291
8. Infante-Rivard C, Esnaola S, Villeneuve JP (1989) Role of endoscopic variceal sclerotherapy in the long-term management of variceal bleeding: a meta-analysis. Gastroenterology (96): 1087–1092
9. Johnston GW, Rodgers HW (1973) A review of 15 years experience in the use of sclerotherapy in the control of bleeding oesophageal varices. Br J Surg (60): 797–800
10. Kiefhaber P, Kiefhaber K, Huber F (1986) Die endoskopisch-therapeutische Anwendung des Neodym-YAG-Lasers im Gastrointestinaltrakt. Neue Techniken in der Medizin. Springer, Berlin Heidelberg New York, pp 25–29

11. Kleber G, Sauerbruch T, Fischer G (1989) Pressure of intraoesophageal varices assessed by fine needle puncture: its relation to endoscopic signs and severity of liver disease in patients with cirrhosis. Gut 30 (2): 228–232
12. Larson AW, Cohen H, Zweibau B (1986) Acute esophageal variceal sclerotherapy. Results of a prospective randomized controlled trial. JAMA 255 (4): 497–500
13. Roussou J, Gonzales-Lavin L, Cosgrove D (1989) A multicenter study: randomized clinical trial of fibrin sealant in patients undergoing resternotomy or reoperation after cardiac operations. Surgery 97: 194–203
14. Scheele J, Stricker KT, Groy RD (1981) Hepatitisrisiko bei der Fibrinklebung in der Allgemeinchirurgie. Med Welt 32: 783–788
15. Scheurlen M, Egberts E-H (1988) Was ist gesichert in der endoskopischen Therapie der oberen Gastrointestinalblutung. Internist 29: 755–764
16. Sivak MV (1985) Sklerotherapie: Stand 1985. Internist 26: 32–42
17. Sugg U (1985) Risiko der Hepatitisübertragung durch humanen Fibrinkleber. Dtsch Med Wochenschr 110: 1161–1162
18. Terblanche J, Krige JE, Bornman PC (1989) The management of oesophageal varices and portal hypertension (editorial). S Afr Med J 75(12): 561–562
19. Wilson RH, Campbell WJ, Spencer A (1989) Rigid endoscopy under general anaesthesia is safe for chronic injection sclerotherapy. Br J Surg 76 (7): 719–721
20. Wördehoff D, Spech HJ (1987) Prophylaktische Ösophagusvarizensklerosierung. Dtsch Med Wochenschr 112 (24): 947–951

# Therapy of Gastrointestinal Fistulas with Fibrin Sealant

M. JUNG, and B. C. MANEGOLD

## Abstract

Gastrointestinal and respiratory fistulas are commonly associated with a prolonged and complicated clinical course. The technique of endoscopic fistula treatment using fibrin tissue adhesives was developed during the past decade. Fibrin sealing can be achieved by endoscopic application of a two-component system (Tissucol) which promotes the normal process of wound healing. The substance was first used in babies in closing isolated hair fistulas and esophageal recurrent fistulas after surgical correction of esophageal atresia. From 1974–1990, 14 babies with recurrent fistulas were treated with Tissucol ($n = 12$) and formerly with Histoacryl ($n = 2$). Endoscopic closure was successful in 11 out of the 14 babies. In two further children endoscopic therapy was successful in gluing broad submucosal lesions in the colonic wall following bougienage and sealing a small perforation in the esophagus following dilatation of a benign stenosis. Since 1984 indication for sealing gastrointestinal and tracheobronchial fistulas in adults has been extended. Esophageal fistulas seem to be a very suitable field for fibrin sealant application. Critically ill patients with anastomotic leakages in the esophagus, perforation due to radiotherapy, trauma, endoscopic procedure, or inflammatory disease were treated as well as patients with tumor fistulas. Endoscopic closures of fistulas were successful in 19 out of 24 patients in one to four sessions. Fibrin sealing failed in nearly all cases of tumor fistulas and in wide infected leakiness. Ineffective results can be caused by incorrect preparation and application of the substance and by early stressing the fibrin clot within the first 24 h. Nevertheless, the endoscopic procedure is especially of interest in critically ill patients and may be today an attractive alternative to major surgical procedures.

## Introduction

Endoscopic sealing techniques to treat fistulas in the alimentary tract are of increasing interest. The objective is no longer the exclusive immobilization of a leakage or perforation up to healing but rather stimulation of active wound closure via the endoscopic approach. Whereas in the past predominantly inorganic sealants were employed for sealing, the main attention now is paid to biological closure of fistulas with highly concentrated fibrinogen. The basic principle of this sealant is simple: the last phase of plasma clotting is imitated with a two-component system (Tissucol). Activation of self-healing is stimulated in the fistular canal, and the exogenous fibrin forms the matrix for this [9, 10]. On the other hand, cyanoacrylate (Histoacryl®, a rapidly polymerizing substance, had only transient clinical significance as an artificial outer clasp for temporary defect sealing [1, 5, 7]. Prolamine sulfate (Ethibloc®), a rapidly hardening mass, has been used to fill a fistular cavity [17].

In endoscopy the technique of fibrin sealing has been adopted from surgical medicine. Whereas the sealant substance is applied in the form of a dense spray over a wide area in surgery, the endoscopic technique is designed for exact punctiform application into and onto the fistular opening. Double lumen catheters guide the separate injections of both components to the surface or to the fistula canal for gluing. Carrier probes with a single lumen also fulfil this function despite the danger of premature precipitation within the probe [8].

## Fibrin Sealant: Properties and Indications

The sealing of fistulas in the digestive tract presupposes the regeneration capacity of the tissue concerned. Since the fibrin clot forms the basis for the areas to be adapted, the surrounding tissue must also be capable of local wound healing. The sealant does not act only as a closing plug for the fistula but also as the substrate for the ingrowth of fibroblasts. The clot is resorbed within 4 weeks and replaced by a connective-tissue scar [10]. Short and fine fistulas with openings which can be well imaged are most suitable for sealing. It is senseless to seal wide defects. Fistulas with a severely damaged epithelium after radiotherapy and fistulas accompanied by chronic infection are also less suitable. Closure is successful in such cases only when sufficient granulation tissue can develop. In the region of infected fistulas, local antibiotic lavages are reported to be helpful [3, 11]. Reports on the sealing of tumor fistulas have been confined to rare cases [18].

The fibrin glue is employed as a two-component system. The two substances fibrinogen and thrombin are mounted in two separate syringes connected by a joint adapter. Depending on the concentration of the thrombin (4 or 500 IU/ml), slow or rapid solidification of the fibrin clot can be attained [16]. However, the concentration employed is probably unimportant. It is important only that the fibrin clot forms in the fistular canal, that it adheres to the tissue, and that premature precipitation in the probe is avoided. Adhesion to the tissue is ensured by prior electrocoagulation of the wound margins or by roughening up with the cytology brush. This deepithelialization seems to be necessary for primary adhesion of the sealant in the fistular canal. Crucial for successful therapy are the first hours after fibrin application since closure of the fistula is initially labile and thus necessitates immobilization of the sealed area. Although about 75 % of the maximum tensile strength is already attained after 3–5 min, i.e., the sealant stability of the human blood coagulum is thus exceeded, tensions should be avoided within the first 24 h [10]. In fistula gluing in the esophagus, the patient is hence given enteral nutrition via a nutrition tube up to final healing. Babies with congenital recurrent esophagotracheal fistulas receive artificial ventilation during the first few days [7, 13]. In patients with sealed bronchial stump breathing gymnastics must be omitted in the following days. Depending on the size of the defect, successful fistula closure may be attained even with a single application [14]. If four or five sealant applications remain ineffective, experience has shown that the therapeutic procedure must be considered [6, 8]. The reason for failure is often an undetected tumor area which does not show a healing reaction to the clot. The fibrin sealant can thus be effective only where it can also induce wound healing. This does indeed restrict its indications.

## Indications and Results

### Congenital Fistulas

Endoscopic therapy of congenital recurrent esophagotracheal fistulas was inaugurated in 1974 by Gdanietz with the report of successful fistula closure using cyanoacrylate [5]. This therapy was afterwards applied successfully in our own patients. Congenital esophagotracheal fistulas are sometimes manifested as rare H fistulas but more frequently as direct connections in congenital esophageal atresia.

Today endoscopic gluing is preferred to surgical reoperation. Cyanoacrylate possesses all the negative properties in this regard connected with synthetic glues. The effect is produced by local foreign body stimulation to wound healing in and around the defect opening. However, the substrate is coughed up again after a few hours or days so that repeated applications are the rule up to definitive closure. In addition, the rapidly precipitating substance leads to damage at the tip of the endoscope [1, 13]. The introduction of the fibrin sealant in this form of treatment simplifies the procedure and the application.

Sealing of congenital tracheoesophageal fistulas is performed under general anesthesia via the rigid bronchoscope. The sealing must be carried out rapidly in 2-min apnea after prior oxygen saturation and continuous control of oxygen saturation. The period up to solidification of the plug is crucial for success. Not more that 1–1.5 ml sealant protein solution is necessary for the often tiny fistular canal located in the dorsal wall of the trachea. Excess substance must be removed immediately to avoid aspiration into the bronchial system. In larger and wider connections between the trachea and esophagus, a "glued-in" cancellous bone implant may facilitate defect closure [5].

From 1977 to January 1990, 14 children with congenital recurrent esophagotracheal fistulas were treated by endoscopic sealing after correction of the esophageal atresia (Table 1). Initially the treatment was carried out with cyanoacrylate ($n = 2$); thereafter, eight children were treated with the fibrin sealant. Definitive wound closure was possible in 11 of 14 cases. Up to final success of therapy, from one to four sealant applications were necessary. Two children had to be reoperated on, and two died of multiple malformations and organ

**Table 1.** Endoscopic fibrin sealing in the gastrointestinal tract: results ($n = 38$)

| Cause of fistula | Upper GI tract | Lower GI tract | Fistula closure | Unsuccessful |
|---|---|---|---|---|
| Congenital | 14[a] | – | 11 | 3 |
| Postoperative | 13 | 2 | 14 | 1 |
| Radiogenic | 3 | – | 2 | 1 |
| Inflammatory | 1 | – | 1 | – |
| Trauma | 1 | – | 1 | – |
| Tumor | 4 | – | 1 | 3 |
| Total | 36 | 2 | 30 | 8 |

[a] $2\times$ Histoacryl.

defects. Years later it is quite possible to verify endoscopically the site of the former fistular formation. This can be recognized as a protruding fold in the upper part of the esophagus.

The sealing of congenital recurrent fistulas can be regarded today as standardized. It is superior to a surgical operation, as a less stressful method. There is agreement that further surgical reinterventions should be discussed only after several unsuccessful sealing attempts.

*Postoperative Fistulas*

Leakages at esophagogastric of esophagojejunal anastomoses after extensive resections are a problem for treatment in the postoperative phase, and these occasionally result in a substantial prolongation of the hospitalization period. Frequently, a tendency to healing cannot be discerned, and the clinical condition stagnates. In 14 of 15 patients with leakages at esophageal anastomoses or with esophageal perforations to the mediastinum and the pleural cavity, and also defects in the lower gastrointestinal tract, the leak was successfully sealed. As a rule, the treatment required from three to five sessions; initially, a tendency to healing was not necessarily visible after the first application of sealant. Nevertheless, healing of the defect was documented in all cases up to 6 weeks after the end of therapy. The concomitant treatment was carried out with nutrition tube and antibiotic cover and with a Bülau drainage in addition in the leakages fistulating into the thorax.

Perforations and fistulas in consequence of surgical endoscopic operations on the esophagus are not unusual. In difficult bougienage of esophageal stenoses or endoprosthesis implantation in benign or malignant stenoses the stability of the esophageal wall is not always predictable. The early diagnosis of a leakage is of eminent importance. Patients with perforations or dehiscences in the non-tumor-bearing esophagus after endoscopic dilation therapy or insertion of a prosthesis were successfully treated in one to four sessions. Endoscopic sealant application was also carried out here immediately after diagnosis (Fig. 1). All lesions healed without problems. Treatments were similarly successful in two patients with inflammatory or traumatic esophageal fistulas. Still in one

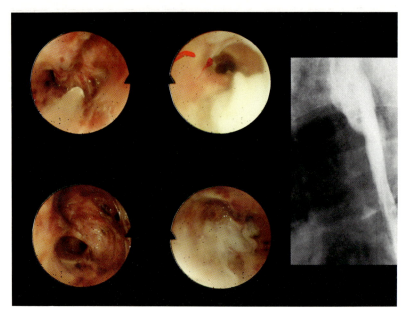

**Fig. 1a–e.** 65-year-old man with cervical esophageal stricture due to caustic injury. **a, b** Broad laceration of the stenotic area and mediastinal perforation after endoscopic bougienage. **c–e** Endoscopic fibrin sealing. Note the white Tissucol clot covering the ruptured esophagus. Complete healing of the damaged esophageal wall in 10 days after two sessions of sealing. No restricture thereafter

patient with persisting leakage after gastrectomy the fistular recurrence was diagnosed 4 months after initial closure.

*Radiogenic Fistulas*

The chances of success in sealing fistulas in the alimentary tract depend mainly on the size of the defect and the regeneration capacity of the tissue lining the lesion. Epithelial damage by radiation fulfills these conditions only with certain limitations. Radiologically induced connections between the esophagus and the trachea are as a rule too extensive to adapt the wound surfaces by fibrin gluing. In addition, local reduction of wall thickness impedes or prevents wound closure. Such fistulas can be adapted best with special endoprostheses, which then ensure perfect sealing. In incomplete fistula closure, mainly at the distal end of the tube, an additional application of fibrin may be advantageous. However, primary sealing is only rarely indicated. We have sealed a radiogenic dorsal defect in the cervical esophagus in only one case. However, the temporary success of therapy was overtaken by progressive tumor growth.

*Tumor Fistulas*

The question as to whether normal wound healing takes place in tumor tissue, and ingrowth of fibroblasts can be induced has not yet been unequivocally answered. Our own experience is negative. Almost all attempts to seal even very tiny tumor fistulas in the esophagotracheal region with fibrin sealant have failed. The clot is vomited out or coughed up completely minutes later, and this occasionally leads to unpleasant aspiration symptoms. While there are reports of successful fibrin sealant application in tumor fistulas, the predominant experience is that the sealant does not adhere to the tumor tissue [6, 18]. We added fibrin sealant in addition to incompletely sealing prosthesis in a patient with a bronchoesophageal fistula in a tumor recurrence at the main bronchus [7, 19]. The operation was successful; however, it remains an open question as to whether the substance encountered normal wound tissue in the marginal zone of the defect.

*Lower Alimentary Tract Fistulas*

Enteroenteral and enterocutaneous fistulas in Crohn's disease should constitute a suitable field for endoscopic fistula therapy with fibrin glue. An entire series of successful applications of sealant is documented in the corresponding literature [3, 11, 21]. The treatment was carried out with elaborate colorectal lavage as well as local lavage, parenteral nutrition, and antibiotics. Local antibiotic lavages are intended to attain a favorable preparation of the fistular lumen for healing. Clear guidelines for the treatment of fistulas in Crohn's disease are not yet available. However, some literature references in this regard are optimistic.

## Discussion

Therapy of local fistulas, leakages, and perforations in the alimentary tract is extended by endoscopic instillation of fibrin sealant ([2, 4, 6, 8, 12] and Costantino et al., this volume). Not only local drying out and immobilization of the lesions but active stimulation of wound healing is required. Application of the fibrin clot is hence not tantamount to "a cork which permanently closes the bottle," but the laying out of a biological matrix which activates the remaining tissue that is capable of regeneration. The question is often posed as to whether spontaneous closure of the leakage is possible over a sufficiently long period, thus rendering endoscopic fistula therapy dispensable; this question cannot be answered in principle. The fact is that the vast majority of patients whom we have treated in severe disease situations were referred by the surgeon himself, and local healing of the defect per se stagnated for an unacceptably long time or did not occur at all. A surgical reoperation had been repeatedly rejected as too stressful [6].

Endoscopic fistula therapy has the unequivocable limits described. The indications for endoscopic sealing in the gastrointestinal and tracheobronchial tracts are as follows:

General: small, tubular defects which can be well visualized and are not connected to the abdominal cavity

Absolute: Postoperative leakage/inflammatory fistulas/instrumental perforations in the esophagus, trachea and bronchus

Relative: Radiogenic defects

Difficult: Chronic, infectious fistulas

Not indicated: Tumor fistulas.

Extensive defects between two organ systems (preferably the trachea and the esophagus) are not suitable for this treatment a priori. Wherever the sealant encounters damaged epithelium (tumor, radiation damage), the fibrin sealant is also of little use.

Main indications for endoscopic sealing are at present postoperative leakages in the esophagus and in the bronchial system after surgical and endoscopic operations [6, 8, 14, 20] and Constantino et al., this volume). Sealant application appears similarly successful in traumatic lesions in these organs. The question as to what extent patients with chronic inflammatory fistular systems in Crohn's disease profit from such a therapy cannot yet be answered. The fundamental preconditions for this are available. Radiogenic defects are appropriate for sealant application only in exceptional cases, and tumor fistulas are also as a rule unsuitable for this treatment. Despite all these restrictions endoscopically applied fibrin sealant has a suitable indication in fistulas in the gastrointestinal tract. Above all, the therapy is of benefit for those severely ill patients for whom other forms of treatment are no longer to be considered.

## References

1. Brands W, Lochbühler H, Raute-Kreinsen U, Joppich I, Schaupp W, Menges HW, Manegold BC (1983) Die Fibrinklebung angeborener Oesophagusmißbildungen. Zentralbl Chir 108: 803–807
2. Cadoni S, Ottonello R, Maxia G, Gemini S, Cocco P (1990) Endoscopic treatment of a duodeno-curaneous fistula with fibrin tissue sealant (Tissucol). Endoscopy 22: 194–195
3. Eimiller A, Berg P, Born P, Barine W, Zellmer R, Neuhaus H, Paul F, Homann H (1989) Fibrin sealing of fistulas in Crohn's disease. In: Waclawiczek HW (ed) Progress in fibrin sealing. Springer, Berlin Heidelberg New York, pp 61–64
4. Eleftheriadis E, Tzartinoglou E, Kotzampassi K, Aletras H (1990) Early endoscopic fibrin sealing of high-output postoperative enterocutaneous fistulas. Acta Chir Scand 156: 625–628
5. Gdanietz K, Wiesner B, Krause I, Mau H, Jung FJ (1974) Gewebekleber zum Verschluß von Oesophagotrachealfisteln bei Kindern. Z Erkr Atmungsorg 141: 46–50
6. Groitl H, Scheele J (1987) Initial experience with endoscopic application of fibrin tissue adhesive in the upper gastrointestinal tract. Surg Endosc 1: 93–97
7. Jung M, Brands W, Manegold BC (1987) Therapeutische Endoskopie mit Fibrinkleber. Med Welt 38: 141–146
8. Jung M, Brands W, Manegold BC (1988) Endoskopische Fisteltherapie mit Fibrinkleber. Schweiz Rundsch Med Prax 77: 3–5
9. Kaeser A, Dum M (1987) Grundlagen der Fibrinklebung-Wirkprinzip- und Infektionssicherheit von Tissucol. Z Herz Thorax Gefäßchir [Suppl] 1: 5–10

10. Kaufner HK (1986) Grundlagen der Fibrinklebung. In: Reifferscheid M (ed) Neue Techniken in der operativen Medizin. Springer, Berlin Heidelberg New York, pp 3–6
11. Kirkegaard P (1982) Treatment of postoperative fistulae with the fibrin-adhesion system Tisseel. In: Tisseel/Tissucol-Symposium: areas of application, problems and perspectives in current surgery. Immuno Scientific Workshop, Scanticon, Aarhus, pp 25–29
12. Kohler B, Köhler G, Riemann JF (1988) Spontaneous esophagotracheal fistula resulting from ulcer in heterotopic gastric mucosa. Gastroenterology 95: 828–830
13. Manegold BC, Lochbühler H, Lochbühler H (1988) Endoskopische Verklebung kongenitaler oesophago-trachealer Rezidivfisteln und Fisteln. In: Manegold BC, Jung M (eds) Fibrinklebung in der Endoskopie. Springer, Berlin Heidelberg New York, pp 28–39
14. Meyer G, Lange H, Wenk H, Schildberg FW (1988) Endoscopic sealing of gastrointestinal fistulae (abstract). Surg Endosc 2: 62
15. Pridun N, Heindl W, Redl H, Schlag G, Machacek E (1986) Animal studies as for the problem of the bronchial fistula. In: Schlag G, Redl H (ed) Thoracic surgery – cardiovascular surgery. Springer, Berlin Heidelberg New York, pp 121–125 (Fibrin sealant in operative medicine, vol 5)
16. Redl H, Schlag G (1986) Fibrin sealant and its modes of application. In: Schlag G, Redl H (eds) Thoracic surgery – cardiovascular surgery. Springer, Berlin Heidelberg New York, pp 121–125 (Fibrin sealant in operative medicine, vol 5)
17. Riemann JF, Ell C (1985) Endoskopischer Verschluß einer tumorbedingten oesophagomediastinalen Fistel mit einer schnellhärtenden Aminosäurelösung. Dtsch Med Wochenschr 110: 396
18. Rolfs HC, Bülzebruck A (1988) Kombinierter therapeutischer Einsatz von Fibrinkleber und Tubusimplantation bei ösophagobronchialen Tumorfisteln. In: Manegold BC, Jung M (eds) Fibrinklebung in der Endoskopie. Springer, Berlin Heidelberg New York, pp 66–68
19. Straumann A, Gyr K, Stalder GA (1984) Tissue adhesive in the prevention of esophageal tube migration: report on a new method. Schweiz Rundschau Med Praxis 73: 1086–1087
20. Waclawiczek HW (1987) Endoskopischer Verschluß infizierter Bronchusstumpf-Fisteln nach Lungenresektion mit der Fibrinklebung (FK) – Klinische und experimentelle Ergebnisse. Z Herz Thorax Gefasschir 1 [Suppl]: 63–66
21. Wenzel M (1985) Fistelverschluß mit Fibrinkleber. Chir Praxis 34: 267–275

# Endoscopic Approaches for Occlusion of Fistulas

V. LANGE, G. MAIWALD, T. SOUVATZI, and G. MEYER

## Abstract

The experience in endoscopic treatment of fistulas gained within a period of more than 10 years is reported. In 117 patients 320 treatments were performed. The overall success rate for occlusion was 72 %. In all patients a two-component glue consisting of thrombin and fibrinogen was used for local fistula treatment, mostly as the one and only drug, sometimes in combination with other substances. Emphasis is placed on unique technique developed 8 years ago, called fistuloscopy, i.e., the percutaneous investigation through the fistular tract. Factors influencing the result of treatment are analyzed. A fistular tract shorter than 1 cm or active Crohn's disease at the site of the fistula cannot be occluded. The success rate is worse the older the fistula and the lower it is localized in the gastrointestinal tract. Endoscopic occlusion of fistulas should be attempted because it never makes a situation worse; however, it can shorten an otherwise long-lasting conservative treatment in about 70 % of patients.

## Introduction

The treatment of fistulas belongs to the everyday duties of the surgeon. Nevertheless this problem is given relatively little attention in the literature. Two reasons may explain this situation. Fistulas occur in the surgical patient population mainly after resections in the gastrointestinal, biliary, or respiratory tract. They are thus the expression of a wound healing disorder and therefore a complication. It is obviously difficult to place the main focus on a lack of success. Under conservative treatment, postoperative fistulas usually heal without sequelae even if this is a long and drawn-out process [9], so that ultimately there is no doubt about the surgical outcome. However, in the past few years there has been an increase in reports of successful occlusion of fistulas with the aid of endoscopy [1, 3, 5, 6, 11]. We report here our own experience with the endoscopic treatment of fistulas which was obtained on a larger number of patients than the series published to date.

## Patients and Methods

From 1987 to 1992 our group performed endoscopic surgery on 117 patients in the surgical departments of two university hospitals (Medical University of Lübeck and Großhadern Hospital, University of Munich), using fibrin glue to treat fistulas. Patients with tumor fistulas, stomalike intestinal fistulas, septic fistulas, and fistulas with obstruction distal to the intestinal fistula opening were excluded from treatment.

Our own techniques of fistula gluing have been described in detail in other publications [7, 8]. The basic rules are repeated here in brief. All fistulas are subject to pretreatment consisting of several days of irrigation. Irrigation is performed with isotonic saline solution, preferably with the addition of fibrinolytic drugs. The irrigation can be conducted manually several times a day or as prolonged irrigation. Before endoscopic therapy radiological imaging of the fistula should be performed, an antibiogram of the fistula secretion should be available, and in the case of colonic fistulas an orthograde intestinal irrigation should be performed, as in colon surgery. At the time of gluing the patient's temperature should have been below 38 °C for at least 24 h. Commercially available gastro-, colo-, recto-, or proctoscopes are used for gluing the fistulas. These are used to adjust to the intestinal opening, and a double-lumen catheter (Duploject) is used for probing. The investigation should preferably be performed with the simultaneous possibility of radioscopy so that contrast medium can be applied for duct imaging if required. Fibrin glue (Tissucol Duo S human fibrinogen, human thrombin, steam treated) is applied through the double-lumen catheter. The aim should be to fill the entire fistula duct with fibrin glue. However, we consider it particularly important to seal the intestinal fistula opening. Wide fistula openings (> endoscope diameter) can be reduced by the intramural injection of fibrin glue with the aid of an endoscopic sclerosis needle. In such cases the glue is inserted in fractionated form (1 ml fibrinogen, 1 ml 0.9 % NaCl, 1 ml thrombin, 1 ml 0.9 % NaCl). Likewise, 1 % polidocanol can be used for this purpose, which also leads to considerable swelling of the mucosa. Before gluing, older fistula ducts or cavities that have formed a glossy pseudoepithelium should be freshened up with a brush or forceps until capillary bleeding occurs. This produces a reactive bed for the glue.

Fistulas of large volumes (gallbladder, small intestine) are treated with adjuvant somatostatin therapy if their volume exceeds 300 ml within 24 h [4]. Patients with fistulas of the upper gastrointestinal tract receive parenteral nutrition for 5 days and those with fistulas of the colon for 7 days. Antibiotic coverage with an appropriately tested antibiotic is provided from the time of gluing up to 1 week after the operation. We monitored fistulas of the upper gastrointestinal tract radiologically or endoscopically; those of the lower gastrointestinal tract were monitored mainly on a clinical basis. A renewed intervention was conducted if fistula secretion recurred prematurely.

Fistula openings that are not accessible to the conventional endoscopic procedures for anatomical reasons are investigated fistuloscopically [8]. This is an endoscopic intervention through the available drainage channel. Broncho-

or gastroscopes are used for this purpose. If the fistula channel is very narrow, bougienage of the duct can be performed under anesthesia and radioscopy. Fistuloscopy is performed under anesthesia at least on the first occasion, while repeat investigations can often be conducted just with analgosedation. Fistuloscopy should be performed only on fistulas that have been present for at least 10 days because the drainage channel is stable enough after this period so that the drainage can be removed and the endoscope inserted into the same channel. A mild insufflation of air through the gastroscope can considerably improve visual coverage. In older fistulas the duct or the cavity does not collapse. Endoscopy using a bronchoscope, which does not permit air insufflation, can also be performed under water by introducing saline solution through the instrument channel. However, the view is normally unsatisfactory due to suspended blood and detritus. In such cases, the bolus-style injection of air through the instrument channel using a large syringe has proved a better option.

In the case of large necrotic cavities it may be sensible to perform débridement endoscopically in the cavity at roughly 2-day intervals. Follow-up management after fistuloscopy is analogous to the directions given above. If a fistulous cavity is present without any connection to the gastrointestinal tract, the patient can be given enteral nutrition again immediately after treatment.

## Results

A total of 117 patients were enrolled in the study for the given observation period to occlude a fistula or an abscess cavity with fibrin glue. Of these, 40 were referred to us for fistula treatment. The treatment was successful in 24 (60%). From our own patient population 77 were treated, 60 with a successful outcome (78%). Six fistulas starting from the trachea, a bronchus, or pulmonary tissue were all occluded, although there was strong selection of the patient population here since bronchial fistulas more than 2 mm in diameter were not treated in this way. The remaining fistulas were localized in the gastrointestinal tract, mediastinum, abdomen, or peritoneum. Of these 111 patients therapy was successful in 78 (66.5%).

Of the 68 patients treated exclusively in the conventional endoscopic way, success was achieved in 49 (72%). We selected fistuloscopy as the only endoscopic access in 37 patients, and 29 of these (78%) could be helped. Twelve patients were treated with a combination of conventional endoscopy and fistuloscopy, with success in six cases (50%).

The age of the fistula and its relation to the outcome of therapy are presented in Table 1. The number of treatments required for lasting fistula occlusion is shown in Table 2. It can be seen from these tables that an increasing fistula duration negatively influences success, and that the chances of success become poorer with an increasing number of interventions. The positive aspect at the end of Table 2 should not hide the fact that the small group of patients treated six or more times represents a selected group which promised a hope of successful treatment (constant decrease in secretion). Patients who showed no tendency to improvement after several interventions were not treated so frequently.

**Table 1.** Fistula duration and outcome of treatment

| Fistula duration | | Success | |
|---|---|---|---|
| | $n$ | $n$ | % |
| 0– 1 week | 8 | 7 | 87 |
| 1– 4 weeks | 55 | 44 | 80 |
| 4– 8 weeks | 29 | 21 | 72 |
| 8–12 weeks | 4 | 3 | 75 |
| 12–26 weeks | 7 | 4 | 57 |
| 26–52 weeks | 6 | 3 | 50 |
| >52 weeks | 8 | 2 | 25 |
| Total | 117 | 84 | 72 |

From the large number of data obtained it is worth highlighting a few points. We found fistulas of the upper gastrointestinal tract in 52 patients and successfully occluded them in 40 (77%). With respect to the lower gastrointestinal tract, this was the case in 27 of 43 patients (63%). Suture insufficiencies were the cause in 68 patients, success being achieved in 52 (76%). Iatrogenic injuries were thought responsible for the fistulas in 12 patients, and the success rate in these cases was 57% (8 patients). Fistulas which we attributed to inflammatory erosion, although sometimes difficult to differentiate from suture insufficiency, were diagnosed in 27 patients, in 20 of whom therapy was successful (74%).

Fistuloscopic investigations were undertaken in a total of 62 patients; 92 fistuloscopies were performed. This is equivalent to nearly one-third of the total of 290 investigations for fistula treatment with fibrin. Table 3 provides information about the fistuloscopic interventions. In nine patients the investigation was terminated as a diagnostic measure because either tumor recurrence was discovered, extensive necroses were present that could not be cleared endoscopically, or there were large necrotic cavities which did not have reactive wall structures, especially in the small pelvis. Thin-caliber gastroscopes were used for fistuloscopy in two-thirds of the cases. The remaining investiga-

**Table 2.** Number of gluings and results

| Number of gluings | | Success | |
|---|---|---|---|
| | $n$ | $n$ | % |
| 1 | 54 | 43 | 80 |
| 2 | 24 | 15 | 62 |
| 3 | 15 | 12 | 80 |
| 4 | 9 | 5 | 55 |
| 5 | 4 | 1 | 25 |
| 6 | 6 | 4 | 75 |
| 7 | 1 | 1 | 100 |
| 8 | 3 | 2 | 75 |
| 10 | 1 | 1 | 100 |
| Total | 117 | 84 | 72 |

**Table 3.** Fistuloscopic measures

| Measure | | Success | |
|---|---|---|---|
| | *n* | *n* | % |
| Débridement/drain | 3 | – | – |
| Gluing | 28 | 20 | 71.5 |
| Débridement and gluing | 22 | 16 | 72.5 |

tions were performed with the bronchoscope, and two cases with a rigid recto-scope. Access for fistuloscopy proved adequate in 48 patients, while a widening of the drainage channel was necessary for investigation in 14 patients, including the diagnostic examination.

No complications from fistula gluing were observed during the conventional investigational approach. We have presented the complications of fistu-loscopy in detail elsewhere [8]. Once the use of the overpressure apparatus for introducing the fibrin glue was discontinued, no further complications occurred during fistuloscopy.

The follow-up of the patient population presented here was performed by questioning the family physicians and patients by telephone, sometimes also as part of follow-up examination in the polyclinic. Fistulas that were not initially occluded and those which recurred within 3 months were classified as unsuc-cessful treatment. This finding was documented for 33 of the 117 patients (28 %). Six patients were lost to follow-up, producing a follow-up rate of 95 %. A recurrence of the fistula occurred after more than 3 months in two patients: a rectovaginal fistula in the case of Crohn's disease after 2 years and a vagino-sacral fistula after rectal extirpation and radiotherapy 12 months after success-ful occlusion. In this case tumor recurrence was detected at the same time. Of the patients observed for a median of 11.6 months 76 can be classified as having a permanently occluded fistula. The median follow-up of only 1 year is due to the fact that about half the patients suffered from a malignant disease and died after progression or recurrence of the basic illness.

The following proved to be particularly unfavorable conditions for fistula occlusion: a fistula duct shorter than 1 cm (success 1/9), combination fistulas which connect more than one hollow organ with a cutaneous opening (4/8), fis-tulas in Crohn's disease (3/11), active Crohn's disease in the area of the fistula not possible to occlude (0/5), and fistulas originating from the pancreas (6/11). A particularly unfavorable situation was a pancreatic duct open-ending in the fistula, which could be occluded in only one of four cases.

## Discussion

The results presented here and the results of other research groups [3, 6, 11] show without doubt that a gastrointestinal fistula can be occluded endoscopi-cally. Nevertheless the discussion of these successful outcomes based on scien-tific criteria is problematic. The polymorphic picture of fistulas makes a classification or grouping virtually impossible. Further factors which encumber a comparative analysis are the duration, varying degree of contamination, localization of the fistulas, and patient's general condition. This large number of different parameters hardly allows a comparative analysis with alternative fistula treatments, such as purely conservative therapy [9] or treatment with gastrointestinal hormones [4]. Neither do the different selection criteria for this therapeutic procedure allow a comparison. In addition to these problems, it could be argued that the fistula may have occluded spontaneously at the time of treatment. A clarification of these questions could be achieved only within an animal experimental study which would have to be performed on large animals to be able to intervene endoscopically.

However, an experienced surgeon can easily tell whether success is attributable to the glue or to a spontaneous course. The definition of successful treatment is: immediate, complete, and permanent elimination of fistula secretion after the last gluing. It is an impressive experience for the attending physician and his patient to have endoscopically achieved such a result in what appear to be hopeless surgical cases. At the same time, the majority of these treatments can ultimately be presented only as case reports due to the polymorphic picture of fistulas.

Our patient population contains a number of cases which we would no longer accept for treatment today after analysis of our data. This includes primarily florid Crohn's disease in the area of the fistula and fistulas less than 1 cm in length. Another group with an extremely poor prognosis are patients who develop a fistula dorsally after anterior resection. If this fistula runs along the blank sacral fascia, there is hardly any reactive tissue available to facilitate rapid healing by fibrin gluing. In such cases, a preternatural anus is virtually unavoidable. Fibrin gluing can be attempted after evacuation of the bowels via a stoma, but in such cases the natural course of fistula healing is hardly influenced by fibrin application.

Finally, the value of fistuloscopy should be stressed emphatically. Cope [2], a Canadian radiologist, was the first to examine fistula ducts with a thin-caliber arthroscope for diagnostic purposes. In addition to the reports of our own experience [8], collected since 1986, reports are now available from two Japanese groups who also used fistuloscopy for assessment and targeted drainage of abscesses and fistulas [10, 12]. We have learned that fistuloscopy can achieve more than simply being a diagnostic and/or drainage measure. Necroses can repeatedly be cleared fistuloscopically, comparable with changing the dressing on a secondarily healing wound. The application of fibrin glue appears to accelerate the cleaning of the base of the wound and stimulate granulation. For this reason we have come to prefer fistuloscopy for fistulas with large cavities even if we can reach the fistula opening by conventional endoscopic means.

## *References*

1. Bianchi A, Solduga C, Ubach M (1988) Percutaneous obliteration of a chronic duodenal fistula. Br J Surg 75: 572
2. Cope C (1988) Needle endoscopy in special procedures. Radiology 168: 353–358
3. Groitl H, Scheele J (1987) Erste Erfahrungen mit der endoskopischen Anwendung eines Fibrinklebers am oberen Gastrointestinaltrakt. Z Herz Thorax Gefasschir I [Suppl 1]: 74–78
4. Grosman I, Simon D (1990) Potential gastrointestinal uses of somatostatin and its synthetic analogue octreoide. Am J Surg 85: 1061–1072
5. Hedelin H, Nilson AE, Teger-Nilsson AC, Thorsen G, Petterson S (1982) Fibrin occlusion of fistulas postoperatively. Surg Gynecol Obstet 154: 366–368
6. Jung M, Schlicker H, Manegold BC (1987) Therapeutische Endoskopie mit Fibrinkleber. Med Welt 38: 141–146
7. Lange V, Meyer G, Wenk H, Schildberg FW (1990) Fistuloscopy – an adjuvant technique for sealing gastrointestinal fistulae. Surg Endosc 4: 212–216
8. Lange V, Meyer G, Schardey HM, Andres HJ (1991) Occlusion of gastrointestinal fistulae by means of endoscopy. ACA 3: 104–108
9. McIntyre PB, Ritchie JK, Hawley PR, Bartram CJ, Lennard-Jones JE (1984) Management of enterocutaneous fistulas: a review of 132 cases. Br J Surg 71: 293–296
10. Nakagawa K, Momono S, Sasacki Y, Furusawa A, Ujiie K (1990) Endoscopic examination for fistula. Endoscopy 22: 115–118
11. Wenzel M (1985) Fistelverschluß mit Fibrinkleber. Chir Praxis 34: 267–271
12. Yamakawa T, Suzuki S, Kobayashi H, Honda S, Ohtaki S, Fukuda N, Amano H, Uno K (1991) Fistuloscopy for the management of postoperative intra-abdominal abscesses. Endoscopy 24: 218–221

# Fistulas in Crohn's Disease as a Complication of the Underlying Disease

A. EIMILLER

## Abstract

Endoscopic fibrin sealing for the occlusion of fistulas in Crohn's disease was first used in 1985 in a young female patient with an active phase of inflammation and a fresh rectovaginal fistula. In the setting of a prospective study 15 more cases of patients with fistulas were treated in this way.

Occlusion of the fistula was achieved in 14 cases. Relapses and complications did not occur, except one abscess 2 months later in one patient. Fistula occlusion by fibrin sealing is an easy and well tolerated method and represents a substantial improvement of therapy of fistulas in Crohn's disease. Neither conservative therapy nor surgical intervention are affected by this method.

## Introduction

According to the literature, early diagnosis and optimized therapy favorably influence the occurrence of complications and the development of the disease [1]. The first aim is to avoid these complications. If fistulas develop, the established measures are conservative therapy (optimized therapy of the basic disease [2], total parenteral nutrition [3], formula diets [4], metromidazole [5], azathioprim of 6-mercaptopurine [6], and possibly cyclosporin [7]) and surgical therapy. In more than 80 % of cases at least a temporary fistula occlusion can be achieved without severe side effects and, thus, an improvement in quality of life by fibrin sealing of the fistula. A remarkable advantage of this method is the absence of interference with the established conservative and surgical methods.

The incidence of Crohn's disease, according to data in the literature, increased from the 1950s to the mid 1970s; in the 1980s it declined again. At present it is between 3 % and 9 % in Western Europa, with the highest incidence in Scandinavia. A fistula as a complication of Crohn's disease develops in more than half of the patients. The published data vary from 10 % to 59 %. According to Kruis et al. [8] the correct figure is around 50 % ; the lower figures are thought to be due to insufficient diagnostic procedures or to too short a period of observation.

The cause of the basic illness is not known, and, consequently, there is no causal therapy. Treatment possibilities involve influencing the local inflammation process. A survey by Allgayer and Kruis [2] shows the effect on the arachidonic acid cascade of established therapeutic medication and substances which could possibly facilitate well-directed therapy in the future. Since there are effective substances for the suppression of the inflammatory processes, our main aim must be a prompt diagnosis of the patients, in order to avoid complications of the prolonged disease. For the fistula this should be possible based on the approach presented by Malchow [1]. Although the occurrence of fistulas according to his definition is in fact a late complication, this incident usually occurs together with an inflammation; the therapeutic decisions at this point are directed toward the basic illness. If possible, complications are handled with minimal interventions.

## Materials and Methods

Endoscopic fibrin sealing was used in 16 cases with fistulas in Crohn's disease in the context of a prospective study carried out at the Gastroenterology Department of the Klinikum Ingolstadt between 1985 and 1989. The follow-up time was at least 6 months in all patients.

Before the deciding on therapy the following steps are necessary:

- Verifying the diagnosis, using the criteria of Lennard-Johns et al. [9]
- Verifying the location and expansion of the inflammation and the fistula
- Assessing inflammation activity, according to Best et al. [10]
- Determining the patient's age
- Evaluating the patient's psychological state.

The procedure for fistula bond includes several steps:

- Draining and reducing the amount of secretion from the fistula using total parenteral nutrition
- Cleaning of the fistula using antiseptic liquids for flushing and brushes for mechanical cleaning
- Degranuling tissue and removing pseudoepithelium in the fistula sinus using brushes or the bare fiber of the laser, according to P. Berlin (personal communication)
- Closing the fistula, starting with a fibrin clot at the luminal end and filling the fistula and injecting in the surrounding tissue step by step
- Avoiding of complications through the administration of metromidazole and intravenous immunoglobulin.

The first fistula occlusion carried out by myself was planned as a minimal intervention. The patient was a young woman with an active phase of inflammation. She had a temperature of 38°–40°C and severe diarrhea. She was suffering from the passage of stool through her vagina. The gynecological consulting examination revealed a rectovaginal fistula and ulcerous vaginitis. The patient's psychological condition was marked by feelings of isolation, and all therapeutic steps were rejected. To stop the passage of stool through the vagina, at least temporarily, and to achieve a positive therapeutic effect and sound relationship between the patient and the attending physician, a fibrin bond of the fistula was carried out. After the fibrin bond the passage of stool through the vagina ceased. At the gynecological control examination 3 weeks later the fistula could no longer be detected. The patient has been relapse-free for 6 years.

This surprisingly positive result was the basis for a pilot study. Two more patients with chronic low-output fistula, one woman with high-output fistula, and 13 patients with an acute attack and formation of new fistula were included in the study. Cases with fox-den-like fistula require a special technique and are not mentioned here.

## Results

Our results to date have been successful closure in 9/9 anorectal fistulas, 4/5 rectovaginal fistulas, 1/1 enteroenteric fistula, and 1/1 enterovesical fistula. No direct complications have been observed. One abscess occurred after 2 months and was healed with a pigtail drainage.

## Discussion

The effectiveness of fistula therapy has by now been confirmed in the literature data for the above conservative methods. With conservative methods only limited improvements are achievable but no cure, according to Fahrländer [11], but even surgical therapy shows disadvantages.

– In the acute inflammatory stage surgical therapy has a negative effect on the general course of the disease.
– Bad scars sometimes form disturbing sphincter function.
– There is a tendency for recrudescence (40%–80%).

In a study with 28 cases of rectovaginal fistula Heyen et al. [12] concluded that most patients needed proctectomy, whereas Radcliffe et al. [13] with 90 cases of rectovaginal fistula recommended that: "Conservative therapy and minor local interventions are the therapy of choice."

The aim of therapy in Crohn's disease is to avoid complications by early diagnosis and early and adapted therapy and follow-up. If patients suffer from fistula, therapy is multimodal. Within the framework of conservative or semi-conservative management of fistula in Crohn's disease, the fibrin bond introduced in 1987 [14] can contribute substantially to improving the quality of life of patients with Crohn's disease.

## References

1. Malchow H (1985) Z Gastroenterol 23
2. Allgayer H, Kruis W (1990) Z Gastroenterol 28: 117–120
3. Greenberg GE et al (1976) Total parenteral nutrition and bowel rest in the management of Crohn's disease. Gut 17: 828

4. Morain C et al (1984) Elemental diet as primary treatment of acute Crohn's disease: a controlled trial. Br Med J 288: 1859
5. Jacbbovits J et al (1984) Metronidazol therapy of Crohn's disease and associated fistulae. Am J Gastroenterol 79: 533
6. Korelitz BJ, Present DH (1985) Favorable effects of mercaptopurine on fistulae of Crohn's disease. Dig Dis Sci 30: 58
7. Hanauer BH, Smith MB (1993) Rapid closure of Crohn's disease fistulas with continuous intravenous cyclosporin A. Am J Gastroenterol 88: 646–649
8. Kruis W, Weinzierl M, Eisenberg J (1979) Dtsch Med Wochenschr 104: 865–867
9. Lennard-Johns et al
10. Best et al
11. Fahrländer H (1984) Dtsch Med Wochenschr 109: 1093
12. Heyen F et al (1989) Dis Colon Rectum 32: 379–383
13. Radcliffe AG et al (1988) Dis Colon Rectum 31: 94–99
14. Eimiller A, Neuhaus H, Paul F (1987) Fortschr Gastroenterol Endosk 17: 60–62

# Technical Description and Results of Endoscopic Treatment of Various Solitary Rectal Ulcer Syndrome Pictures

A. EDERLE, G. BULIGHIN, S. PILATI, and S. DESIDERI

## Abstract

Solitary rectal ulcer syndrome is a rare disease producing different pictures, such as superficial ulcers, deep and large ulcers with elevated margins, and polypoid formations modifying the architecture of the rectum. The medical and surgical treatment usually suggested reduces symptoms but gives only partial results on the lesions. We have tried to treat this syndrome ulcers with Tissucol using the colonscope. We applied the product on small ulcers and both injected and applied it on large and elevated ulcers. Four-lumen catheter or sclerotherapy needles were used. Rapidly solidifying Tissucol was used for application and slowly solidifying Tissucol for injection. Two groups (1 and 2) of six patients each were treated both with dietetic and hygienic measures; group 1 was also treated with an application of Tissucol. After 15 days all six ulcers were healed in group 1 and none in group 2. After 1 year no ulcer was present in group 1 and 3/6 in group 2. Five patients with large elevated ulcers sometimes with multiple polypoid formations and with partial stenosis were treated as described above. Good results on symptoms were obtained in all patients. Complete healing was obtained in 3/5 patients and partial healing in 2/5 patients. However, the rectal lesions of these two patients were probably due to tuberculosis and endometriosis, rather than to solitary rectal ulcer syndrome.

## Introduction

Solitary rectal ulcer syndrome is a rare disease; its pathogenesis is likely to be associated with impaired anorectal dynamics leading to localized ischemic phenomena [1, 2]. The ulcer is generally located 5–15 cm from the anal edge. In most cases a prolapse of varying kind and degree is present [3, 8]. From a morphological point of view the disease is characterized not only by ulcer lesions [1, 4], and the following different pictures may be found (with the percentages in our series of 66 patients):

a single (12.1 %) or multiple (12.1 %) flat ulcer,
a single (16.6 %) or multiple (3 %) raised margin ulcer,

a single polyp (7.5 %),
confluent polypoid formations (3 %), and
minimal alterations (nodular mucosa and/or erosions, petechiae, localized hyperemia; 51.5 %).

Flat ulcers are generally smaller in size (< 1 cm) whereas those with raised margins are usually larger and may be associated with or superimposed on polypoid lesions, which can be so extended as to create a certain stenosis of the rectum. Symptoms are generally not very marked when minimal lesions or small and superficial ulcers are present (mostly rectorrhage) but are more so in the presence of large ulcers or widespread polypoid lesions (rectorrhage, tenesmus, proctalgia, mucorrhage, etc.).

Patients usually benefit from hygienic-dietary measures (high-fiber diet, correct evacuating position, etc.) [9], but the evolution of the lesion does not seem to be influenced by these measures. The various pharmacological attempts seem to yield similar results, while some authors report more encouraging results using particular surgical techniques for prolapse correction [10]. However, this kind of surgery can be suggested only for some of these patients, it is not easily performed, and it is not free of complications.

For some time we have been investigating the effectiveness of endoscopic treatment with a human fibrin sealant (Tissucol) both on the ulcer lesion and on the symptoms related to this syndrome [11]. Human fibrin sealant has been employed for some time in surgery and has recently been introduced in endoscopy due to its sealing, hemostatic, and angiogenic properties and to its ability to stimulate fibrogenesis and tissue regeneration. In particular, in endoscopy it has been used for the scarring of esophageal ulcers secondary to varices sclerosis, on bleeding ulcers, and for closing fistulas [12, 13]. It also seems to foster scarring of peptic ulcers [14].

## Materials and Methods

The results of our previous studies have shown that it is appropriate to divide the cases into those with small (< 1.2 cm), superficial ulcers and those with large ulcers associated with growing lesions. In our experience, the former respond well to the applicative technique but the latter only to the joint injective-applicative technique.

We treated seven patients with small superficial ulcers with the applicative technique alone. Six of these (group 1) were compared with the same number of non endoscopically treated patients, similar in terms of kind of lesion, age, and sex (group 2). All the patients followed the hygienic-dietary measures described above. An endoscopic check was carried out at 15 days and at 1 year.

We treated five cases of large ulcers, some associated with polypoid formations, with the injective-applicative technique. In three of these patients we began using only the applicative technique, but due to unsatisfactory results after two or three sessions we switched to the injective-applicative technique. Due to the small number of these cases we were not able to compare them with a control group, nor did we establish to follow up the patients and to repeat the treatment if necessary.

Generally these patients were treated every 15 days until the ulcer disappeared. They were checked according to the speed of response to treatment, extent of the lesion, and symptoms. Mean follow-up time was 19 months.

Tissucol is made up of lyophilized human plasma clotting proteins dissolved in a solution containing aprotinin and of lyophilized bovine thrombin dissolved in a solution of calcium chloride. Different thrombin concentrations produce different speeds of solidification of the constituents. In endoscopy Tissucol can be either applied or injected. In the former case we insert through the channel of the endoscope a multichannel catheter that allows us to mix the constituents at the site of application, and with it we apply rapidly solidifying fibrin sealant. When we inject, we use a double needle or a normal esophageal varices sclerosis needle and inject slowly solidifying fibrin sealant.

In the applicative technique once the catheter has emerged from the tip of endoscope we first try with a small amount of the sealant to see where it falls. This enables us to choose the highest point so that Tissucol can spread over all the lesion, creating a single mass that then retracts. This mass adheres very well and stabilizes within a few hours. For our own convenience we color the sealant with methylene blue.

In the joint injective-applicative technique, in most cases we use a normal sclerosis needle to inject 0.5–1.0 ml slowly solidifying Tissucol at each injection, especially at the margins of the lesion and in no case on the necrotic tissue. This provides adhesion to the margins where there is reactive epithelial hyperplasia on which the sealant can more easily carry out its scarring and tissue regenerative action. In addition, when injected through the mucosa, it can prevent the mucosa itself from slipping on the underlying planes, likely the main pathogenetic mechanism in this disease. The quantity to be injected is about 2–5 ml per session; the exact quantity, however, depends on the extent of the lesion. The injection probably also helps to anchor the fibrin sealant. At this stage we procede to applying Tissucol using the multichannel catheter. The applied Tissucol adheres better in the presence of injected sealant, which is in part located also on top of the lesion thus creating a single more stable and more adherent mass.

Polypoid lesions are cut with a loop as much as possible, and when necessary Tissucol is then applied on the polypectomy site. When a partial stenosis is present, we dilate it using a balloon.

## Results

### Small and Superficial Ulcers

At the endoscopic check carried out 15 days after the beginning of treatment we found that all the patients treated only with hygienic-dietary measures still had an active ulcer lesion. On the other hand, all the patients treated with applied Tissucol plus hygienic-dietary measures had completely scarred ulcers ($p < 0.004$). At 1 year only three patients of six in the group treated only with hygienic-dietary measures showed at endoscopy a healed ulcer lesion. In the other group the ulcer was still scarred in all six patients.

## Large Ulcers at Times with Polypoid Formations

In one case of an ulcer with a diameter of more than 2 cm and with raised margins located on a very congested fold we obtained a progressive and then complete reepithelialization of the ulcer after four sessions, with a 15-day interval between them. At the check 7 months later treatment had to be repeated because of a relapse of an ulcer of about 1.3 cm, which was no longer present at the following check 1 year later.

In another patient in whom multiple sessile formations up to more than 2 cm in diameter with widespread ulcer lesions were present in the area 5–14 cm from the anal channel we obtained scarring of the ulcer lesions and a reduction in polypoid formations after five sessions during which Tissucol was injected and applied, and the polypoid lesions were cut as much as possible with a loop. For 2 years the patient has now been checked about every 6 months without true ulcers being found; however, growth of the polypoid formations at times with erosions was present. These formations have been removed each time.

In a third patient in whom a raised margin ulcer of about 2 cm was present we obtained only a slight reduction in the ulcer after four sessions. The patient was in the meantime found to be affected by tuberculosis, which may have been responsible for the rectal disease.

In a fourth case fibrotic folds were present all around the distal 4–6 cm to the rectum, significantly reducing its diameter. Most of the surface of these folds had ulcer lesions. The patient had been operated upon a few years earlier because of pelvic endometriosis, probably responsible for the fibrotic process and the lesions that we found. After several sessions of injective and applicative treatment and of dilatation with a balloon associated with removal by a loop of the polypoid formations, the ulcer process had reduced to a diameter of less than 1 cm without, however, disappearing completely but spreading for a period of 8 months when no treatment was carried out.

In the last patient, who came to us because of marked rectorrhage and mucorrhage, we found a double ulcer lesion (of 1.5 and 0.5 cm) on a marked and congested fold. After three sessions the smaller ulcer disappeared completely, and the diameter of the larger one was very much reduced. Later, due to complete lack of symptoms, the patient refused to return for check-ups. After 1 year he is still asymptomatic.

All the five patients reported that symptoms had either completely disappeared or were constantly reduced.

## Discussion

Although our comparison in small and superficial ulcers was not randomized, it does confirm that human fibrin sealant is useful in the treatment of the solitary rectal ulcer syndrome. When evaluating the disappearance of the ulcer in the two groups one must also consider the varying time of the macroscopic pictures of solitary rectal ulcer syndrome. It is well known that this is a chronic disease with a natural history lasting years, but with pictures and lesions that change with time.

The modification of the mucosa when an ulcer is present is made up of a solution of continuity with a reactive epithelial hyperplasia particularly visible on the margins. The fibrin sealant probably acts on this regenerative mechanism, thus contributing to lasting epithelial regeneration. Considering also that the likely pathogenesis of the solitary rectal ulcer is associated with local ischemia [1, 2], the angiogenetic effect of the fibrin sealant may also play a role. It is probably a mechanism that is similar to that of the scarring of venous ulcers of the lower limbs, in which Tissucol has been successfully used for years.

The results that we obtained in the few cases of large ulcers with polypoid formations are quite different. In these patients we obtained partial results only by combining the injective and applicative techniques. The injection of Tissucol on the margins of the lesion probably has the advantage of better anchoring the fibrin sealant, which produces a more stable and long-lasting complex. We cannot exclude that the submucosal injection may have a more marked angiogenetic action and may act more favorably on the regenerative mechanism by working on non necrotic tissue and may contribute to reducing the slipping of the mucosa on the underlying planes, thus acting on one of the hypothetical pathogenetic mechanisms of this lesion.

Our results were positive in three cases as for scarring of the ulcer for relatively long periods, although the syndrome was obviously still present, and were only partial in two cases, in which another disease was present to which the rectal lesions were probably secondary. We refer to the case with tuberculosis and to that with rectal fibrosis probably secondary to endometriosis in which there is a marked alteration of the rectum. Obviously in these cases no treatment can solve the problem, and there was no indication for surgery. In all the patients symptoms disappeared or were markedly reduced, which justifies the treatment, whether scarring is obtained or not.

Before definitely suggesting this kind of treatment, various technical aspects such as the timing and the number of applications must be investigated in more depth, and the technique must be more completely established. The technique for the use of fibrin sealant is not particularly time-consuming or complicated, since it requires minimum staff training and a maximum of 5 min to prepare the various components. Bearing in mind the poor results yielded by the most commonly employed kinds of treatment, we believe that fibrin sealant may in the future acquire a fundamental role in the treatment of the solitary rectal ulcer syndrome.

## References

1. Rutter KRP, Riddel RH (1975) The solitary ulcer syndrome of the rectum. Clin Gastroenterol 4: 505–530
2. Rutter KRP (1974) Electromyographic changes in certain pelvic floor abnormalities. Proc R Soc Med 67: 53–56
3. Keigley MRB, Shoulder P (1984) Clinical and manometric features of the solitary rectal ulcer syndrome. Dis Colon Rectum 27: 507–512

4. Martin CJ, Parks TG, Biggart JD (1981) Solitary rectal ulcer syndrome in Northern Ireland, 1971–1980. Br J Surg 68: 744–747
5. Ford MJ, Anderson JR, Gilmour HM, Holt S, Sircus W, Heading RC (1983) Clinical spectrum of "solitary ulcer" of the rectum. Gastroenterology 84: 1533–1540
6. Womack NR, Williams NR, Holmfield JHM, Morrison JFB (1987) Pressure and prolapse – the cause of solitary rectal ulceration. Gut 28: 1228–1233
7. Melange M, Vanheuverzwyn R, Mathieu P, Detry R, Heuchamps Y, Haot J, Dire C (1985) L'ulcere solitaire du rectum: un syndrome. Acta Gastroenterol Belg 48, 2: 140–147
8. Schweiger M, Alexander Williams J (1977) Solitary rectal ulcer syndrome of the rectum – its association with occult rectal prolapse. Lancet 2: 1228–1233
9. Van Der Brand-Gradel V, Huibregtse K, Tytgat GNJ (1984) Treatment of solitary rectal ulcer syndrome with high fiber diet abstention of straining at defecation. Dig Dis Sci 29: 1005–1008
10. Nicholls RJ, Simson JNL (1986) Anteroposterior rectopexy in the treatment of solitary rectal ulcer syndrome without overt rectal prolapse. Br J Surg 73: 222–224
11. Ederle A, Bulighin G, Scattolini C, Novelli P, Negri S, Ferrari C, Vantini I (1988) La sindrome dell'ulcera solitaria del retto: diagnosi, terapia e follow up. Atti II Congresso Italiano di Colonproctologia, Padova, pp 749–754
12. Costantino V, Pedrazzoli S, Miotto D, Pescarini L (1985) Trattamento delle fistole con l'uso di colla di fibrina umana (Tissucol). Risultati preliminari della nostra esperienza. Acta Chir Ital 41: 756–760
13. Ederle A, Bulighin G, Orlandi PG, Pilati S, D'Agostino U, Sipala G (1991) Trattamento endoscopico di fistole gastroenteriche mediante colla di fibrina. Atti del X Congresso Nazionale dell'Associazione Italiana Gastroenterologi Ospedalieri. Monduzzi, Geneva, pp 385–388
14. Ederle A, Scattolini C, Bulighin G, Benini L, Orlandi PG, Talamini G, Vantini I (1991) Does the combination of a human fibrin sealant with ranitidine accelerate the healing of duodenal ulcer? Ital J Gastroenterol 23: 354–356

# The Occlusion of Anal Fistulas in Crohn's Disease

N. WOLF, I. SCHNEIDER, K. THALER, and C. SCHNEIDER

## Abstract

Surgical treatment of anal fistulas occurring in Crohn's disease is often precluded by the specific conditions of the underlying disorder. The use of fibrin for the successful treatment of esophageal and bronchial fistulas encouraged us to start a clinical trial on the occlusion of Crohn's fistulas by fibrin adhesive.

In a pilot study nine patients suffering from Crohn's disease were treated with tissue sealant to occlude anal fistulas. After curettage and cleaning we injected up to 3 ml fibrin adhesive into the fistulas. This procedure was repeated to a maximum of 17 injections over several months.

Complete healing was achieved in three cases. In two cases, a distinct clinical improvement could be noticed. The remaining four patients did not show any improvement. Considering the simplicity of this therapeutic approach we feel that occlusion of perianal fistulas in patients with Crohn's disease is a valuable alternative to surgical excision.

## Introduction

When considering the treatment of anal fistulas in Crohn's disease, it is necessary to keep in mind the etiology and the special features of these fistulas. The perianal fistulas in Crohn's disease are the result of an infection conveyed through minute breaches of the lining of the anal canal or along an anal gland. The inflammation is further promoted by infectious bowel contents [6]. This view is also supported by other authors [1, 2]. Radcliffe emphasizes the penetrating nature of Crohn's disease for the genesis of perianal fistulas. Recurrent inflammation as well as a delayed and often complicated healing with resulting incontinence limits the aggressiveness of operative therapy. For this reason we were trying to find a different therapeutic approach. The promising results reported after the application of fibrin adhesives in treating bronchial or esophageal fistulas [4, 8] encouraged us to start a clinical trial on the occlusion of Crohn's fistulas by fibrin adhesive.

## Material and Methods

Two men and seven women were treated between April 1988 and March 1989. Patients' ages ranged between 24 and 37 years. Three patients had bowel resections in their previous history, and four others had a defunctioning colostomy or ileostomy before treatment with tissue sealant. Based on the activity of their Crohn's disease all patients received anti-inflammatory drugs, corticosteroids, or antibiotics during therapy. Before the application of fibrin glue all fistulas were carefully probed, curettaged, and cleaned by the injection of NaCl 0.9 %. Depending on the extent of the perianal fistulas up to 3 ml fibrin adhesive was instilled. This procedure was repeated at short-term intervals up to 17 times over several months.

## Results

We achieved complete healing in three cases. Occlusion always occurred very promptly, i.e., only a few applications of the adhesive were necessary to close the fistula. When more than three sessions were needed, complete healing was never obtained. A distinct clinical improvement was verified in two cases. In one patient who had multiple tracks we saw a closure of part of the fistulas. The other patient, with one large fistula, showed a distinct reduction in size. In both cases a diminution in fistulous discharge was noted. The remaining four patients showed no amelioration by the sealing therapy. Neither undesired side effects nor any complications were seen in our patients.

## Discussion

Before speaking about the surgical therapy in Crohn's fistulas it is necessary to know that the most important precondition for therapeutic success is sufficient medical treatment of the inflammatory bowel disease [3]. Because of delayed healing and the risk of resulting incontinence a more conservative approach to surgical therapy in Crohn's fistulas should be used, as reported by Tuxen and Castro [7], Stelzner [6] and Stein [5]. In view of this requirement the concept of sealing appears promising. Unlike fistulas of other causes, those in Crohn's disease usually have no epithelial lining which must be removed prior to occlusion therapy as it would interfere with leukocyte reaction and prevent the formation of connective tissue. In spite of the small number of patients included in our series it is evident that the chance of complete healing is inversely proportional to the number of sealant applications. A defunctioning ileo- or colostomy seems to have a positive influence on the progress of healing. In addition to the systemic medication we used local anti-inflammatory preparations such as Colifoam and Betnesol for further reduction in the local inflammatory reaction. Based on our findings we feel that occlusion of fistulas in Crohn's disease by fibrin adhesive is a valuable therapeutic alternative.

## *References*

1. Buchmann P (1988) Lehrbuch der Proktologie, 2nd edn. Huber, Bern, pp 82–97
2. Eisenhammer S (1958) A new approach to the anorectal fistulous abscess based on the high intermuscular lesion. Surg Gynecol Obstet 106: 595
3. Gladisch R (1988) Fibrinklebung von Fisteln bei Morbus Crohn – Kommentar: In: Manegold BC (ed) Fibrinklebung in der Endoskopie. Springer, Berlin Heidelberg New York, p 167
4. Jung M (1988) Verklebung von Fisteln am Ösophagus. In: Manegold BC (ed) Fibrinklebung in der Endoskopie. Springer, Berlin Heidelberg New York, pp 48–54
5. Stein E (1986) Proktologie – Lehrbuch und Atlas. Springer, Berlin Heidelberg New York, pp 279–294
6. Stelzner F (1981) Die anorektalen Fisteln, 3rd edn. Springer, Berlin Heidelberg New York, pp 44–223
7. Tuxen PA, Castro AF (1979) Rectovaginal fistula in Crohn's disease. Dis Colon Rectum 22: 58–62
8. Waclawiczek HW (1988) Der endoskopische Verschluß infizierter Bronchusstumpffisteln nach Lungenresektion mit der Fibrinklebung. In: Manegold BC (ed) Fibrinklebung in der Endoskopie. Springer, Berlin Heidelberg New York, pp 17–22

# Human Fibrin Sealants and Postoperative Fistulas: 25 Cases

V. Costantino, A. Alfano D'Andrea, and S. Pedrazzoli

## Abstract

Human fibrin sealant was used to accelerate the healing process in a total of 25 fistulas: 9 intestinal, 2 biliary, 1 vaginal, and 13 pancreatic. All patients received adequate nutritional support, and their secretions were reduced by pharmacological treatment. They underwent repeated X-ray check-ups to achieve a proper positioning of the drainages and to control the healing process. As soon as the fistulas showed a regular tract and a low outflow, they were treated with fibrin sealant. Quick and stable healing was obtained in 22 cases. In three patients we obtained only a reduction of secretions and lumen.

## Introduction

Fistulas are frequent and life-threatening complications of abdominal surgery. They prolong hospitalization and therefore entail an individual and social cost. Precise operative techniques and full preoperative correction of nourishment needs are considered useful in preventing fistulas.

Post-operative fistulas can be divided into "early" and "delayed" fistulas. Early fistulas (before the sixth or seventh postoperative day) are usually due to errors in surgical technique. This kind of fistula does not benefit from the physiological adhesions which occur after all operations, and its secretions spread into the abdominal cavity. These fistulas are associated with a high mortality rate and frequently require second-look surgery ranging from simple suture of the leaking anastomosis or local drainage to wide surgical demolitions. Delayed fistulas (after the seventh postoperative day) are more common and benefit from the physiological scarring of the organism. They usually require only conservative treatment consisting of purely medical treatment, sometimes associated with interventional radiology, for example:

- Fasting with total parenteral nutrition and sufficient caloric intake for the patient's condition and for the postoperative catabolic phase with the target of reducing physiological secretions
- Almost complete pharmacological suppression of pancreatic, intestinal, and biliary secretions, using somatostatin or analogues

- Prevention and treatment of septic complications with antibiotic prophylaxis or, in the case of positive cultures, specific antibiotic therapy
- Compensation of losses and general restabilization of the patient
- Washings, to clean the fistula and to buffer secretions
- Protection of the skin against aggressive secretions, especially pancreatic and biliary secretions
- X-ray check-up to the fistula's shape and the position of the drainages for removing the secretions as quickly and directly as possible [1, 2]

We believe that the latter morphological aspect is very important since it is the goal of all conservative therapies. The initial morphological aspect of fistulas may influence their healing, depending on whether the path is simple and straight or complex and ramified with unadequately drained side sacs requiring further radiological and surgical maneuvers to achieve good drainage. The presence or absence of drainages, their position in relation to the fistula, type of fistula (pancreatic, jejunal etc.), and the possible occurrence of septic or hemorrhagic complications can also influence healing as well as the fistula's outflow [1, 2].

In treating the fistulas that we observed we used all the above conservative methods to obtain a low-outflow straight fistula with sufficiently a small lumen to be sealed with fibrin glue.

## Materials and Methods

Since October 1983 we have treated 25 patients with fibrin sealant. Two further patients were excluded from further treatment and underwent surgery: a woman previously treated for a perirectal abscess drained through the rectum, who had a presacral intestinal cyst and a man affected by a ramified perineal fistula. Both of these patients underwent surgery. The 25 patients were as follows: One had vaginal fistula after hysterectomy and Hartmann's operation due to cancer of the rectum. Nine had intestinal fistulas, one after Kock's reservoir ileostomy due to inflammatory bowel disease, one gastrocutaneous fistula after pancreatic pseudocyst marsupialization, one following external biliary drainage, four fistulas, one esophagojejunostomy after total gastrectomy due to gastric cancer, two with fistula after left colectomy due to rectum cancer. Thirteen had pancreatic fistulas: six after pancreaticoduodenectomy (two for pancreatic cancer, two for ampullary cancer, and two for endocrine tumors), two after left pancreatectomy (one for chronic pancreatitis, one for cystoadenoma) one after excision of an insulinoma in the head of the pancreas and three after surgical treatment of acute necrotizing pancreatitis (one after percutaneous drainage of a pseudocyst, one necrosectomy and drainage, one cystojejunostomy). Two had biliary-cutaneous fistulas after atypical right hepatectomy for hepatic echinococcosis.

The first patient treated was affected by a vaginal fistula after Hartmann's operation and was kept on conservative therapy for over 1 year with no benefit. All patients underwent fistulography for detecting the diameter, length, and source of the fistula: if necessary, the drainage was repositioned under radiological control [3]. If the fistolous tract was grossly linear, the fibrin sealant (rapid reconstitution) was prepared and injected through a radiopaque double-lumen catheter. Under fluoroscopic control, the glue was applied as close as possible to the origin of the fistulous tract. In some cases a hydrosoluble radiopaque medium was added to the sealant to control the point of glue application under fluoroscopic view. In all patients the repositioning of the drainage was performed under radiological control. The patients with gastrointestinal, pancreatic, or biliary fistulas underwent complete parenteral nutrition with functional exclusion of the intestinal tract affected by the fistula.

## Results

Of 13 patients with pancreatic fistulas 10 required only one sealant application, which completely and definitively cured the fistula with no complication. In three patients, each of whom had previously received pancreaticoduodenectomy for pancreatic cancer, only a reduction in the fistula's outflow and lumen were achieved. One week later the sealant was successfully applied for the second time in all three patients. In six of nine patients with enteric fistulas the pathology resolved completely with a single application of the sealant. The treatment was unsuccessful in two patients with enteric fistulas: one who had had gastrotomy during surgery for marsupialization of a pancreatic pseudocyst 10 years earlier and one who had had Kock's ileostomy after total colectomy due to inflammatory disease.

One patient who developed a fistula on esophagojejunostomy after total gastrectomy died 1 week after sealing for massive intestinal infarction. Both biliary fistulas and the vaginal fistula were successfully treated with fibrin sealant.

## Discussion

Fistulas may appear after abdominal surgery. They can be classified not only according to their etiology but also according to the nature of their secretion and flow. A generally accepted treatment is total parenteral nutrition, pharmacological suppression of secretions, antibiotic therapy, and drainage procedures. X-ray examination is essential to evaluate the effectiveness of treatment: when healing cannot be achieved quickly by medical treatment drainage procedures are mandatory to make the fistulous tract smooth and straight enough so that all secretions as well as the injected washing fluids or contrast media can be easily aspirated through the catheter. If collateral branches or cavities are detected, additional catheters must be positioned. Only at this time can fibrin sealant treatment be helpful; earlier use is not likely to be effective, while delayed treatment is useless because late healing could occur anyway with no time gain.

The use of fibrin sealant is beneficial since it forms a physiological barrier against organic secretions. It is self-shaping, and its pressure prevents the outflow of secretions through the fistula, diverting them through their natural channels. When the obstructive effect of the sealant ceases with the end of the antifibrinolytic action of the aprotinin and degradation of the thrombin, new granulation tissue has grown to close the fistula. In our experience, no local or general infection and no allergic reaction or other complications possibly due to the presence of the glue were observed. The technique has proven simple and easy to repeat. In some cases which would otherwise have required a surgical treatment sealing shortened the healing time. The savings in time and diminution in risk justify the comparatively high cost of the sealant. Although the number of patients who have received this treatment is still low, the results are satisfactory and encouraging for the future.

## *References*

1. Costantino V, Petrin P, Pasquali C, Liessi G, Pedrazzoli S (1992) Use of fibrin sealant in the treatment of pancreatic fistulas. In: Pederzoli P (ed) Pancreatic fistulas. Springer, Berlin Heidelberg New York, pp 201–210
2. Costantino V, Pedrazzoli S, Miotto D, Pescarini L (1985) Trattamento delle fistole con l'uso della colla di fibrina umana (Tissucol), risultati preliminari della nostra esperienza. Acta Chir Ital 41: 756–760
3. Miotto D, Feltrin GP, Costantino V, Petrin P, Pedrazzoli S, Chiesura M (1985) Riposizionamento e completamento dei drenaggi chirurgici addominali. Chir Triv XXV (1): 83–86

# Fibrin Sealant in Endoscopic Gynecological Surgery

J. F. H. GAUWERKY

## *Introduction*

Fibrin sealing has become an accepted tool in many fields of surgery. In many areas fibrin sealing has superseded conventional surgical techniques, increased postoperative safety, and even made possible new therapeutic approaches. In the light of endoscopic surgery fibrin glue has a certain place in the therapy of interstitial fistulas, ulcera, and bleedings. I am sure that fibrin glue in operative gynecological endoscopy will also be of increasing interest for the following indications: for wound closure, as a substitute for conventional sutures; to achieve hemostasis and control bleeding; and for prophylaxis of adhesions. In the present paper I report our experience with fibrin glue in endoscopic myomectomy, tubal anastomosis, and the endoscopic construction of neovagina.

## *Endoscopic Myomectomy*

### *Operative Technique*

The preparation is performed with classical endoscopic instruments, grasping forceps, and scissors, depending on the presentation of the myoma. The various steps of preparation are demonstrated in Fig. 1. The capsula of the myoma is transsected with scissors or electrosurgically (Fig. 1b). Thereafter the myoma is grasped with grasping forceps and removed step by step in the same way as in the classical transabdominal approach. The wound of the uterus (Fig. 1c) is closed with interrupted or continuous sutures. The wound is covered with fibrin glue (Tissucol Duo S, human fibrinogen, human thrombin, steam treated; Fig. 1d) to reduce bleeding from the wound edges and for prophylaxis of adhesions.

### *Results*

Figure 2 demonstrates the increasing number of uterus-conserving operations and the increasing number of endoscopic procedures. Table 1 compares the results of our endoscopic procedures with those in laparotomy. It can be seen

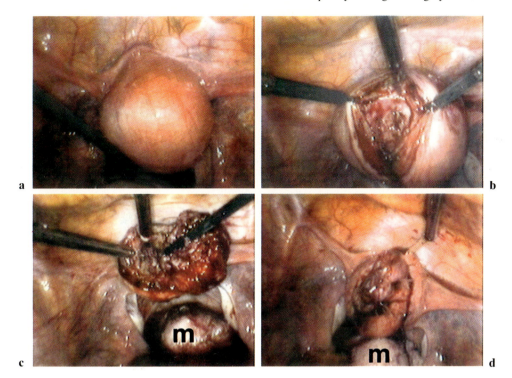

**Fig. 1a–d.** Principle of endoscopic myomectomy. **a** Myoma located at the fundus of the uterus. **b** Incision of the capsula and preparation with classical instruments. **c** The myoma is removed. **d** The uterine wall has been closed with interrupted sutures and the wound is covered with fibrin glue

that the number and the diameter of the laparoscopically removed myomas is a somewhat smaller than those removed by laparotomy. The mean operating time of the endoscopic procedures is slightly longer, but the hospital stay for laparoscopically operated patients – of main benefit to the patient and also of socioeconomic value – is significantly lower. We now perform this procedure on an outpatient basis in selected cases. In my opinion the use of fibrin glue is an adjuvant to improve safety in these cases.

**Table 1.** Results of myomectomy by laparotomy and laparoscopy

|                      | Laparotomy | Laparoscopy |
|----------------------|------------|-------------|
| Diameter (cm)        | 6.9        | 5.1         |
| No. of fibromas      | 2.5        | 1.8         |
| Operation time (min) | 75         | 86          |
| Hospital stay (days) | 11.6       | 4.5         |
| Pregnancy rate       | 50%        | 37%         |

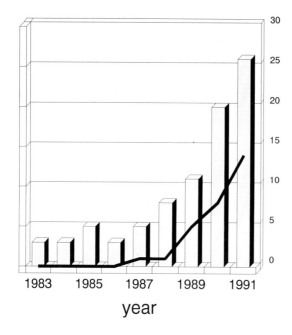

**Fig. 2.** Number of uterus conserving and endoscopically performed operations at the University of Heidelberg. *Bars*, total; *curve*, endoscopies

## Tubal Anastomosis

### Operative Technique

The operative technique corresponds to that earlier published [1]. Preparation of the tubal stumps corresponds to that in laparotomy and microsurgery. After preparation of the tubal stumps a splint is inserted, and the anastomosis is performed with fibrin glue over the inlaying splint as a guide. The anastomosis is secured by an 6-0 vicryl seromuscular suture placed at the antimesenteric border at the 12 o'clock position (Fig. 3).

### Results

**Animal Experiments.** In animal experiments on rabbits I have demonstrated that tubal anastomosis with fibrin glue is as effective as the conventional microsurgical technique [1]. This is true for isthmic anastomoses, ampullary anastomoses, and anastomoses after resection of tubal segments (Fig. 4). Also the healing of glued anastomoses in the isthmic region is similar to the microsutured anastomoses [3] (Fig. 5). These good results made possible the first clinical application in cases of sterilization and request for reversal.

**Clinical Study.** Until now we have operated on 13 patients with this new technique (Table 2). Six patients became pregnant (a pregnancy rate of 46%);

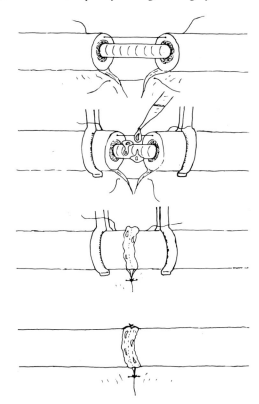

**Fig. 3.** Principle of endoscopic tubal anastomosis with fibrin glue

**Table 2.** Results of endoscopically performed tubal anastomoses

| Patient no. | Age | Patency | Pregnancy |
|---|---|---|---|
| 1 | 37 | + | 2× abortion, LPD |
| 2 | 25 | + | Term pregnancy |
| 3 | 38 | + | Term pregnancy |
| 4 | 39 | + | No, LPD |
| 5 | 35 | 2 MS | Term pregnancy |
| 6 | 41 | + | No, LPD |
| 7 | 30 | + | EUG |
| | | 2 MS | Recurrent EUG contralateral |
| 8 | 36 | ? | No |
| 9 | 33 | ? | No |
| 10 | 34 | ? | No |
| 11 | 37 | − | Dehiscence |
| | | 2 MS | Term pregnancy |
| 12 | 38 | ? | No |
| 13 | 26 | ? | No |
| 14 | 32 | + | Intrauterine pregnancy |

2 MS, second microsurgery; LPD, luteal phase deficiency; EUP, extrauterine pregnancy.

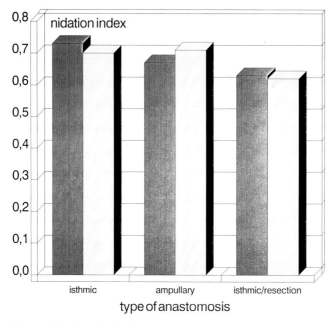

**Fig. 4.** Results of tubal anastomoses with fibrin glue *(dark bars)* compared to microsurgical techniques *(light bars)* in rabbits. Nidation index in isthmic, ampullary, and isthmic anastomoses with resection of tubal segments

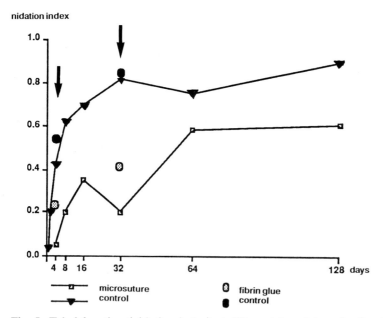

**Fig. 5.** Tubal function (nidation index) at different time intervals after isthmic anastomoses performed microsurgically and with fibrin glue *(arrows)*

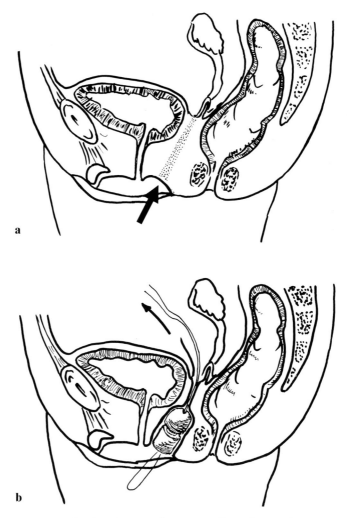

**Fig. 6a.** Cross-section of the pelvis in the absence of a vagina. *Dotted area*, the space between bladder and rectum, where a vagina is to be created (modified according to Vecchietti [5]). **b** Principle of the Vecchietti method: creation of a vagina by continuous pressure to the interlabial space. The pressure is induced by tension threads connected with an olive and passing through the space between bladder and rectum to the abdominal wall

there were four intrauterine and two ectopic pregnancies. The first patient operated on had had three intrauterine abortions; a septated uterus, which we corrected hysteroscopically after the first abortion, may have been reason in this case. The ectopic pregnancies occurred in both cases in the anastomosed tube. The anastomoses were patent, as confirmed by ascending hydropertubation during laparoscopy. Comparison of these results of a small group, operated on endoscopically only on one side, with these results attainable by microsurgery, may be somewhat disappointing after the initial enthusiasm. However, I believe that it is possible to further improve the technique of endoscopic tubal anastomoses.

### Endoscopically Assisted Neovagina

#### Operative Technique

The principle of this method is the creation of a vagina by pressure of a mould which is connected with tension threads to the interlabial space (Fig. 6). In this way a vagina is created within 7–14 days. The technique has been reported earlier [4, 5] and is repeated only briefly here (Fig. 7). The uterovesical peritoneum or, in patients with an absent or rudimentary uterus, the pouch of Douglas is opened endoscopically by electrosurgical means or with scissors; a tunnel is then prepared between the bladder and rectum. The tension threads are then passed with a straight needle from the vaginal stump through the prepared tunnel into the abdominal cavity. On each side a separate small cutaneous incision is made at the point at which the tension threads are to be pulled out through the abdominal wall. A large curved needle is inserted into this small incision and guided retroperitoneally to the peritoneal incision under endoscopic control. Each thread in turn is passed through the eye of the curved needle, pulled through to the abdominal wall, and connected with the tension apparatus. The peritoneum is closed with several interrupted sutures or, if appropriate, with fibrin glue.

#### Results

The results of these endoscopically performed neovaginas are summarized in Table 3. Two patients had a testicular feminization, five a Mayer-Rokitansky-Küster syndrome, and in one case a colpectomy was performed during operation for cancer of the cervix. All operations were performed without complications. The functional results were good, with long vaginas.

**Table 3.** Results of endoscopically assisted reconstruction of a vagina

| Patient no. | Age (years) | Indication | Length of vagina (cm) |
|---|---|---|---|
| 1 | 17 | Test. femin. | 8 |
| 2 | 16 | Test. femin. | 12 |
| 3 | 16 | MRK | 10 |
| 4 | 18 | MRK | 11 |
| 5 | 35 | Colpectomy | 8 |
| 6 | 20 | MRK | 12 |
| 7 | 18 | MRK | 10 |
| 8 | 17 | MRK | 8 |

Test. femin., testicular feminization; MRK, Mayer-Rokitansky-Kuster syndrome.

## *Abstract*

According to our results and experience in endoscopic gynecological surgery, fibrin glue is a most helpful adjuvant. The application is very simple; fibrin glue has an excellent hemostatic effect and replaces conventional and technically difficult endoscopic sutures. The adhesion-protecting effect of fibrin glue is still being discussed [6], but there is some clinical evidence, also from our small number of laparoscopically reevaluated patients, that fibrin glue provides formation of adhesions in many cases.

## *References*

1. Gauwerky JFH (1991) Endoskopische Refertilisierung. Zentralbl Gynakol 113: 865–868
2. Gauwerky JFH, Klose RP, Vierneisel P, Bastert G (1992) Fibrin glue for reanastomosis of the fallopian tube – adhesions and fertility. Hum Reproduct 7: 1274–1277
3. Gauwerky JFH, Vetter H, Bastert G (1992) Funktionelle Aspekte der Heilung von mikrochirurgischen Tubenanastomosen – experimentelle Untersuchungen an der Kaninchentube. Zentralbl Gynakol 114: 450–454
4. Gauwerky JFH, Wallwiener D, Bastert G (1992) An endoscopically assisted technique for construction of a neovagina. Arch Gynecol Obstet 252: 59–63
5. Gauwerky JFH, Wallwiener D, Bastert G (1993) Die endoskopisch assistierte Anlage einer Neovagina – operative Technik und erste Erfahrungen. Geburtsh Frauenheilkd 53: 261–264
6. Gauwerky JFH, Mann J, Bastert G (1990) The effect of fibrin glue and peritoneal grafts in the prevention of intraperitoneal adhesions. Arch Gynecol 247: 161–166

# Fibrin Sealing in Endoscopic Surgery

D. WALLWIENER, S. RIMBACH, D. POLLMANN, W. STOLZ,
J. F. H. GAUWERKY, and G. BASTERT

## Abstract

The special merits of fibrin sealing are the possibility of simple atraumatic tissue union and hemostasis and, thus, decreased duration of surgical intervention. This technique is therefore already well established for a number of indications in surgical gynecologic endoscopy. These include, in particular, the reshaping of an ovary after extirpation of a cyst, the application during tubal anastomosis, and the sealing of iatrogenic perforations of the uterus. Unequivocal evidence of the efficacy of fibrin sealing of serous and peritoneal defects with the purpose of adhesion prophylaxis is not yet available. Whereas fibrin sealing due to its good long-term results is regarded as the preferred method for the first-mentioned indications, further studies with a large number of cases and long follow-up are necessary to enable a final evaluation of this technique for the latter indications. No complications were evident in the postoperative course or during follow-up in the 75 laparoscopic fibrin sealings carried out to date. In addition to its wound healing properties, fibrin sealing was found to be intraoperatively superior as the time-consuming endoscopic sutures were replaced in a simple and atraumatic manner; furthermore, a simultaneous hemostyptic action was attained.

## Introduction

Since the introduction of the laparoscopic technique, most of the many reconstructive or organ-preserving interventions in the tubo-ovarian functional unit, adhesiolyses, and surgical treatments of endometriosis in the internal genitals are performed in the gynecology department without an abdominal section being necessary [1].

The use of fibrin sealant has improved a preparation technique which had already been optimized, especially through the employment of lasers and modern high-frequency electrosurgical operation techniques. Fibrin sealant (Tissucol Duo S, human fibrinogen, human thrombin, steam treated) is used for three specific goals: sealing of wound edges and surfaces, attaining a local hemostatic effect, and adhesion prophylaxis by sealing of peritoneal and serous defects, the efficacy of which has, however, not yet been unequivocally ascertained. The basic advantages of fibrin sealant are its exceptional histocompatibility, absorbability, high elasticity, and adhesive strength even in a damp environment.

## Method

The principle of fibrin sealing is based on the last phase of hemostasis. We use a two-component fibrin sealant which is composed essentially of highly concentrated human fibrinogen and a highly concentrated thrombin solution. Solidification begins within seconds of application and is almost entirely completed within a few minutes. It is applied using a cannula when focal or small surface sealing is necessary. Only a thin layer of sealant ought to be applied when larger surfaces are being treated as the time necessary for absorption and final wound healing are highly dependent on the thickness of this layer.

The range of indications for which fibrin sealing is used are discussed in detail below:

Established indications
   Ovary shaping after extirpation of cyst ($n = 26$)
   Local hemostasis (e.g., after myoma enucleation)
   Laparoscopic sealing of artificial perforations of the uterus ($n = 3$)

Indications under study conditions
   Laparoscopic linear salpingotomy ($n = 17$)
   Laparoscopic refertilization ($n = 12$)
   Sealing of serous and peritoneal damage after extensive adhesiolysis (e.g., sealing of intestinal serous damage; $n = 20$)

**Ovarian Cyst Extirpation and Reshaping of Ovaries.** In a large number of patients benign ovarian cysts can be extirpated and the organs preserved without an abdominal section being necessary (Fig. 1). By means of laparoscopic intervention the ovarian capsule is initially incised prior to partially sharp and partially blunt extirpation of the cyst or endometrioma. The resultant damage, which can be sealed using fibrin sealant after hemostasis, leads to the reshaping of the ovary and its surface. This is a technically uncomplicated yet extremely effective method of surgical intervention which we have performed successfully in 26 cases. Ultrasonographic follow-up examinations and a few second-look laparoscopies have revealed no pathological alterations in the newly shaped ovary.

**Laparoscopic Linear Salpingotomy in Isthmoampullary Tubal Pregnancy.** During organ-preserving laparoscopic treatment of a tubal pregnancy by means of linear salpingotomy one is confronted with the problem of closing the wound after the removal of the gestational product. An adaptation of the wound edges and closure of the lumen by means of fibrin sealing are a simple and quick alternative to the time-consuming and difficult endoscopic suture (Fig. 2) and permit to avoid the risk of fistulization in wide-open salpingotomy wound

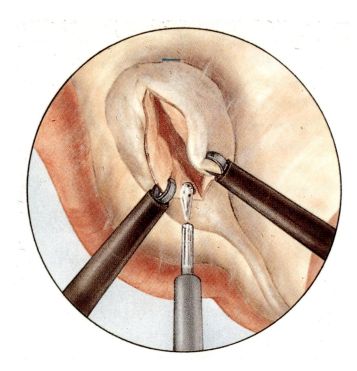

**Fig. 1.** Ovary shaping using fibrin sealant after organ-preserving extirpation of an ovarian cyst

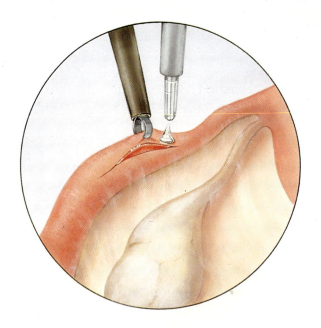

**Fig. 2.** Fibrin sealing of a linear salpingotomy due to an isthmoampullary tubal pregnancy

edges. In 17 cases treated in this manner no difficulties arose intraoperatively due to the use of fibrin sealant. The follow-up examinations showed that the intervention was successful in terms of organ-preserving reconstruction. Two repeat laparoscopies due to extrauterine pregnancies on the contralateral side confirmed this. A fistula was discernible in two patients, albeit after an extremely large tubal pregnancy necessitating a 3-cm salpingotomy in both cases.

**Laparoscopic Refertilization.** A combination of suture and sealing technique is particularly suitable after endoscopic refertilization with end-to-end anastomosis of the tubal stumps. The intratubal splint can be hysteroscopically inserted and placed under laparoscopic control. Fibrin sealant is applied after approximation of the stumps by means of a suture.

**Areal Sealing for Hemostatic Purposes and Reparation of Peritoneal Damage.** A further use of fibrin sealant is in hemostatic areal sealing or reparation of damage. In such cases the bleeding surfaces must first be rinsed with a warm saline solution using a water purifier. The hemostatic effect is promoted by intra-abdominal hypertension with the aid of an insufflator. After laser or electrocoagulation fibrin sealant is sprayed onto a surface as blood dry as possible to attain a permanent hemostatic and sealing effect. The same technique is used for sealing of peritoneal or serous damage in expectation of reattaining the physiologic gliding of the parietal and visceral peritoneal surfaces. Iatrogenic uterine perforations are sealed in the same manner; fibrin sealant is capable of preventing ascending infections as well as primary or secondary hemorrhaging from the damaged surface. A laparoscopic suture is not necessary after fibrin sealing. The uterus must be held in place for 3–5 min until the final fixation of the sealant; an adaptation layer of sealant is applied and this then coated with a fixation layer. Fibrin sealant was used in 15 cases to seal peritoneal damage, in 5 cases of serous damage in the intestinal area, and in 3 cases of uterine perforation. In a few isolated cases second-look laparoscopy was performed during which almost no postoperative adhesions were discerned. The postoperative course was free of complications in every case. Whether the fibrin sealing resulted in significant adhesion prophylaxis must, however, be further investigated.

## Discussion

One may conclude that the use of fibrin sealant with surgical laparoscopic techniques represents a perfection of the minimally invasive preparation concept, which has already been optimized by the use of laser and high-frequency electrosurgical techniques. Fibrin sealing results in a reduction in operation time and simplifies the entire surgical procedure as it is possible to do without complicated endoscopic sutures in many cases [1, 5, 8].

One must emphasize that fibrin sealing leads to physiologic tissue union. However, compared with sutures a higher price must be accepted in the cost versus benefit analysis. The use of fibrin sealant for ovary shaping after extirpation of cysts, for local hemostasis (e.g., after myoma enucleation) and for laparoscopic sealing of iatrogenic perforations of the uterus can be regarded as established indications, while its application in tubal anastomosis for refertilization purposes has been shown to be an extremely successful procedure [2, 3, 6, 7]. However, the technique of fibrin sealing in organ-preserving surgical treatment of tubal pregnancy by means of salpingotomy must be carried out under test conditions until a large enough number of cases has been treated before a final evaluation may be made. This is also true for the application of fibrin sealant to cover serous and peritoneal damage after extensive adhesiolysis and surgical intervention in the tubo-ovarian functional unit. The protective effect, i.e., the avoidance of readhesions, is still under discussion. On the one hand, verification of the absolute necessity of covering damage, particularly after laser preparation, is still lacking. On the other, the effectiveness of the sealing of such damage can be established only by means of second-look laparoscopies, the execution of which is problematic for ethical reasons [4].

Careful consideration is necessary for every intended application of fibrin sealant as far as the cost versus benefit factor is concerned. To what extent the shortening of operation time compensates for this disadvantage must be decided individually for each case. The use of fibrin sealant in gynecologic laparoscopy is, however, extremely promising as far as the established range of indications under discussion and the distinctly advantageous long-term results attained in surgical laparoscopy are concerned.

The advantages of fibrin sealing are:
– Shortened operation time
– Physiologic tissue union and sealing of damage
– Atraumatic operation technique
– Easy handling
– Adhesion prophylaxis

The disadvantages of fibrin sealing are:
– More expensive than suture material
– Necessity of sealing peritoneal damage, particularly after laser preparation unclarified
– Little experience to date and insufficient follow-up to enable final evaluation

A final evaluation is, however, to be left to comparative studies which are more extensive than the pilot study presented here; a long follow-up and a sufficient number of cases are imperative.

## References

1. Wallwiener D, Pollmann D, Gauwerky J, Stolz W, Rimbach S, Bastert G (1992) Suture-free tissue sealing: fibrin glue? In: Bastert G, Wallwiener D (eds) Laser in gynecology. Possibilities and limitations. Springer Verlag, Berlin Heidelberg New York, pp 175–182
2. Baumann R, Volk M, Taubert H-D, Rücker KJ (1987) Refertilisierung beim Menschen unter zusätzlicher Anwendung von Fibrinkleber. In: Kubli F, Schmidt W, Gauwerky J (eds) Fibrinklebung in der Frauenheilkunde und Geburtshilfe. Springer, Berlin Heidelberg New York, pp 73–80
3. Gauwerky J, Forssmann WG, Kubli F (1987) Fibrinklebung versus Nahtanastomose: Experimentelle Untersuchungen zur mikrochirurgischen Refertilisierung. In: Kubli F, Schmidt W, Gauwerky J (eds) Fibrinklebung in der Frauenheilkunde und Geburtshilfe. Springer, Berlin Heidelberg New York, pp 61–68
4. Larsson B, Fianu S, Jonasson A, Rodriquez-Martinez H, Hedström CG, Thorgirsson T (1987) The use of Tisseel (Tissucol) – a two-component fibrin sealant – in operations for fertility as a sealant and for prevention of adhesions: an experimental study and a preliminary clinical evaluation. In: Schlag G, Redl H (eds) Gynaecology and obstetrics – urology. Springer, Berlin Heidelberg New York, pp 90–94 (Fibrin sealant in operative medicine, vol 3)
5. Riss P, Spernol R, Beck A, Schindler K (1986) The use of fibrin glue in experimental tubal surgery. In: Schlag G, Redl H (eds) Gynaecology and obstetrics – urology. Springer, Berlin Heidelberg New York, pp 84–89 (Fibrin sealant in operative medicine, vol 3)
6. Scheidel PH, Wallwiener D, Wiedemann RA, Hepp H (1982) Experimental anastomosis of the rabbit fallopian tube using fibrin glue. Fertil Steril 38: 471–474
7. Wallwiener D (1982) Experimentelle Anastomose-Technik mit Fibrinkleber an der Kaninchentube. Inauguraldissertation, University of the Saarland
8. Wallwiener D (1990) Fibrinkleber in der operativen Laparoskopie. Med Report 13/14

# Endoscopic Modification of the Marshall-Marchetti-Krantz Operation

D. WALLWIENER, S. RIMBACH, E. M. GRISCHKE, J. JANKY, and G. BASTERT

## Abstract

For operative therapy of urinary stress incontinence the Marshall-Marchetti-Krantz operation has proven successful in up to 80 % of cases. With the modifications according to Hirsch (altered suturing technique) and Stolz (all sutures replaced by fibrin sealant), the perioperative complication rate has been markedly reduced. The authors present a new endoscopic modification of the Marshall-Marchetti-Krantz operation, which maintains the principle of vesicourethral suspension using fibrin sealant but avoids extensive incision into the abdominal wall. Based on the concept of minimally invasive surgery, it is replaced by retziusscopy and endoscopic preparation of the cavum retzii.

## Introduction

The Marshall-Marchetti-Krantz (MMK [4]) operation has proven successful for the operative therapy of urinary stress incontinence and has become established as a routine procedure. The principle of the MMK operation consists in vesicourethral suspension performed to restore the descending neck of the bladder to its original intra-abdominal position. To prevent the occurrence of osteomyelites and periostites, Hirsch [2] modified this method; he avoided sutures for fixation to the symphysis but performed suspension of the vaginal fasciae by suturing to the obturator fascia and the tendinous portion of the obturator muscle instead (MMKH operation). Stolz [6] pointed out the risk of splitting sutures with consecutive bleedings as well as complications due to unphysiologic distortion of the anterior vaginal wall and further modified the procedure by replacing all sutures by fibrin sealing. As far as the correction of urinary stress incontinence is concerned, the clinical and urodynamic results achieved by this technique were as good as those achieved with the original method; however, at the same time the complication rate was reduced. The MMKH operation modified according to Stolz has proven an excellent procedure for the operative therapy of urinary stress incontinence, with a success rate of 60 %–80 %. Nevertheless, in view of the minimally invasive techniques constantly gaining ground in gynecologic surgery, the necessity of opening the cavum retzii by Pfannenstiel's incision must be regarded as a drawback of this method.

The authors therefore present an endoscopic modification of the operative technique using "retziusscopy", by which extensive incision into the abdominal wall can be avoided.

## Operative Procedure and Results

Following proper positioning and disinfection, a 1-cm suprasymphysial median cutaneous incision is made. The fascia is partly exposed and also incised. The cone trocar is bluntly advanced into the cavum retzii. Gas-tight closure of fascia and skin is achieved by suturing to the trocar; subsequently, a pneumocavum is created by $CO_2$ insufflation. Distension of the cavum retzii can be observed visually. Visualization of the cavum retzii is achieved by $CO_2$ pressure alone without further manipulation. For extensive preparation of the paraurethral and the retrosymphysial areas a preparation swab is introduced through the working canal of the endoscope and pushed to the obturator and vaginal fasciae. Fatty tissue is carefully removed from the periosteum of the posterior symphysial wall and from the fasciae of the anterior vaginal wall and the neck of the bladder. Prior to preparation individual vessels are coagulated by means of bipolar coagulation to permit exposure of the preparation surface and the tissue layers and avoid hemorrhages obstructing the surgeon's view. Subsequently, the anterior vaginal wall is digitally elevated and, simultaneously, 2 ml fibrin sealant (Tissucol Duo S, human fibrinogen, human thrombin, steam treated) is applied paraurethrally to each side, right and left. The vagina is digitally pressed against the retrosymphysial area for 5–7 min until the fibrin sealant has solidified. Compression is maintained for 24 h by means of a vaginal tamponade. After application of fibrin sealant and compression the pneumocavum is gradually deflated, and the trocar is removed immediately after closure of the cavum retzii. Subsequently, the fascial sutures are tied. Before closing the cutaneous incision a suprapubic catheter is introduced.

The duration of the operation is markedly reduced by avoiding extensive opening and, later, closure of the layers of the abdominal wall. From a technical point of view, direct colposuspension with fibrin sealant is performed analogously to the conventional MMK method without suspension sutures. Accordingly, the postoperative results of the anatomical correction equal those achieved by the conventional procedure. The success of the anatomical correction has been verified by perineal sonography of the reconstructed urethrovesical angle.

## Discussion

In patients with urinary stress incontinence II or III, which cannot be satisfactorily controlled by conservative therapy, the MMK operation has proven a successful procedure by which urinary continence can be restored in 60%–80% of cases [4]. The modifications introduced by Hirsch [2] and Stolz

[6] maintain the principle of vesicourethral suspension but reduce the complication rate by avoiding periosteal sutures for fixation to the retrosymphysial space and replacing all sutures by fibrin sealing, respectively.

The criteria of success of the operation are first of all the subjective indications made by the patients concerning the subsidence of incontinence complaints [7] but also objectifiable parameters of urodynamic function and the results of gynecologic examinations and perineal sonography for control of the anatomical substrate for correction of the descent of the bladder neck.

Regarding topographic and functional results and reduction of the rate of suture-associated postoperative complications the MMK procedure can hardly be essentially improved, in particular after the inclusion of fibrin sealant. After the example of numerous successful applications in various fields of operative surgery [1, 3, 5], also in the MMK operation sealing has taken the place of fixation sutures, which had frequently caused inflammatory complications affecting the periosteum and the symphysial bone of hemorrhages and hematoma formation due to splitting sutures.

From a technical point of view, the application of fibrin sealant through a double-lumen catheter is an uncomplicated procedure well suited for the modified procedure presented in this paper for the first time, which – being an endoscopic technique – is in accordance with the principle of minimally invasive surgery.

During the endoscopic MMK operation the abdomen is not opened, but a $CO_2$ pneumocavus is created and retziusscopy performed. While the endoscopic operative procedure is unproblematic and presents no drawbacks compared to the conventional one, this technique offers the essential advantages of minimally invasive surgery. Trauma inflicted to the abdominal wall is minimalized, the wound healing phase is considerably shortened, and associated postoperative complaints are essentially reduced. Moreover, the cosmetic results are markedly improved.

In conclusion, we consider the endoscopic modification using fibrin sealant to be a further optimization of the MMK operation, particularly with respect to the improvement of perioperative subjective complaints and the reduction of complications associated with the conventional extensive incision into the abdominal wall. Retziusscopy permits endoscopic visualization without the necessity of opening the abdominal wall and offers all the advantages of a minimally invasive surgical technique. While we have been concerned mainly with the operative technique, future work will have to present the results of follow-ups of sufficiently large numbers of patients to establish whether the long-term results differ from those achieved with the conventional procedure, which, however, is not to be expected from the present point of view.

## References

1. Gluckert K, Tesch HJ, Weseloch GK (1984) Fibrinklebung bei Sehnenläsionen – experimentelle Ergebnisse und klinische Aspekte. In: Scheele J (ed) Fibrinklebung. Springer, Berlin Heidelberg New York, p 221

2. Hirsch HA (1979) Über eine neue Modifikation der vesikourethralen Suspension. Arch Gynecol 228: 326
3. Kubli F, Schmidt W, Gauwerky J (1987) Fibrinklebung in der Frauenheilkunde und Geburtshilfe. Springer, Berlin Heidelberg New York
4. Marshall KF, Marchetti AA, Krantz KE (1949) The correction of stress incontinence by simple vesicourethral suspension. Surg Gynecol Obstet 88: 509
5. Melchior H (1985) Fibrinklebung in der Urologie. Springer, Berlin Heidelberg New York
6. Stolz W, Brandner P, Dory F, Bastert G (1989) Marshall-Marchetti-Krantz-Operation mit Fibrinklebung. Geburtshilfe Frauenheilkd 49: 564
7. Stolz W, Schüssler B, Hanke R (1985) Harninkontinenz und Leidensdruck. Arch Gynecol 238: 469

# Minimally Invasive Lung Surgery: Preliminary Results

W. Wayand, R. Woisetschläger, and R. Rieger

## Abstract

From June 1991 to April 1992 we carried out wedge resections of the lung with a minimally invasive technique in 15 patients. The indications were spontaneous pneumothorax in six cases, tumors in five, and systemic diseases in four. In every case the pathological lesion diagnosed preoperatively by X-ray and computed tomography was dealt with without complications. The minimally invasive atypical pulmonary resection is a relatively atraumatic method for peripherally situated pulmonary lesions.

## Introduction

Based on experience gained with more than 1000 laparoscopic procedures over the past 2 years the era of minimal invasive lung surgery became inevitable. The benefits for envisaged patients having minimal invasive surgery compared to conventional surgery were in regard to pain, mobilization, and pulmonary function; in addition, cosmetic results should also be more beneficial after lung surgery avoiding thoracotomy. The most important further technological development in this context was an endoscopically applicable clip suturing device, enabling immediate airtight occlusion of a resection site on the lungs. In the past 9 months we performed minimally invasive thorax surgery in 15 patients for treatment of pathological lesions in the periphery of the lungs [5]. This contribution reports our experience.

## Technique

The operation is carried out under general anesthesia using a double-lumen tube in the usual position on the side, as in posterolateral thoracotomy. An instrument table for immediate performance of a thoracotomy which may be necessary is available in a stand-by position. After washing and draping, the trocars are placed as follows. An 11-mm incision is made for the endoscope in the region of the middle axillary line at the level of the sixth IS. Thoracocentesis with the Veress needle is carried out via this incision. $CO_2$ insufflation such

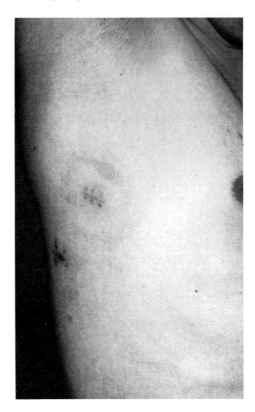

**Fig. 1.** Minimally invasive lung surgery
6 weeks postoperative

as in laparoscopy is not necessary. An aspiration and slurp test confirms the intrathoracic position and thus a free pleural cleft. The endoscope is then introduced by means of the 11-mm trocar. Then under visual control a 5-mm incision about 10 cm laterodorsal to the first incision is made, two intercostal spaces higher for an atraumatic gripping forceps, and in the same IS anterior axillary line. Finally, a 12-mm incision is made for the application of the endogastrointestinal anastomosis stapling device. (This can also be used as a holding forceps without actuation of the clip mechanism, so that a further fixation forceps can generally be dispensed with.)

As shown in Fig. 1 (3 weeks after the operation), the placement of the trocars results in an equilateral triangle with about 10-cm-long sides and standing on one of its apices. Any detachment of adhesions, exploration, and confirmation of the diagnosis is now carried out under visual control. Even pathological lesions just under the surface can be visualized well by blunt expression of residual air from the noninflated pulmonary parenchyma. The part of the lungs to be resected is drawn into the open mouth of the endo-GIA with the fixation forceps and the instrument is discharged. Depending on the extent of the pathological lesion, the instrument (which cuts between a sixfold row of sutures 3.0 cm long) needs to be applied one to eight times. For recovery of the resected tissue it is advisable to introduce the preparation intrathoracically into a plastic bag and to recover it. In two of our own cases a slight enlargement of the incision (patient numbers 12 and 14) was necessary.

Afterwards, the thorax cavity is inspected once more, and a check is made as to whether the row of clips is leakproof after unblocking the tube. A thorax drain is placed under visual control, and the operation is completed after wound closure.

## Patients and Results

Our 15 operations were undertaken on 12 men and 3 women (27–78 years old). The indication was pneumothorax in six cases (five recurrences, one constricted thorax which could not be treated conservatively). In five cases the indication was peripheral round foci (an intraoperative rapid section investigation was carried out in patients 11, 13, 14; if a carcinoma was present, we carried out thoracotomy and lobectomy with lymph node dissection). The overall condition of patient number 12 (78 years old, retired colleague with coronary heart disease in whom percutaneous transluminal coronary angioplasty had been carried out twice) precluded radical antitumor therapy (Figs. 2, 3). Systemic diseases were the indication in four cases (confirmation of diagnoses; suspicion of sarcoidosis and silicosis).

Table 1 presents a description of the patients. In the first patient the clip suture device was not yet available to us in June 1991. The thoracoscopic dissection of the bulla was carried out with the method described by Takeno [12]. It remains a matter of speculation as to whether the raised temperature lasting 3 days was connected with the perhaps not 100% leakproof occlusion of the resulting parenchymal defect.

In patient number 12 (who also ran a fever for 4 days after the operation), the resection dimensions of $8 \times 8 \times 4$ cm probably reached the maximum extent of an atypical wedge resection of the lung. All patients were extubated

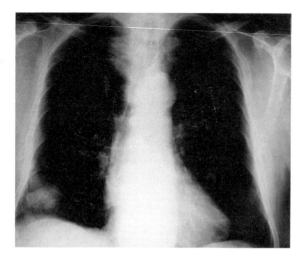

**Fig. 2.** Adenocarcinoma, right lower lobe (patient no. 12)

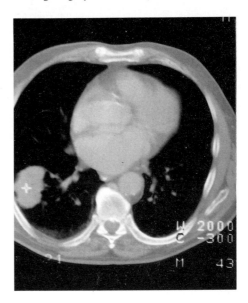

**Fig. 3.** Adenocarcinoma, computed tomography (patient no. 12)

after 12 h at the most. The thorax drains were removed on the 3rd–5th post-operative day in all patients. All patients recovered from the operation without problems, and their wounds healed per primam. On the basis of laparoscopic experience in 650 cholecystectomies in the meantime it was simple for us to apply the technique; the duration of the operations (which were documented in detail) was between 30 and 75 min.

## Discussion

Thoracoscopy has been known for decades. On the basis of the research of Jacobäus, in particular the Austrians Kux, Sattler and Wittmoser are to be regarded as pioneers [4,6, 9,10, 14]. This division of endoscopy has unfortunately been neglected by surgeons. However, atraumatic procedures may be presumed to have those major advantages already known to be associated with laparoscopy (minimization of trauma in its effects on subjective well being, mobilization, and convalescence). It may thus be hoped that such procedures will become rapidly accepted among surgeons. We developed diagnostic thoracoscopy further to enable thoracoscopic lung surgery (this application has hardly been mentioned so far in the literature) for the following indications:

**Pneumothorax.** In all six patients a morphological substrate was demonstrated preoperatively with computed tomography and X-ray, and this was confirmed intraoperatively. If an unequivocal cause of the pneumothorax is not found, a parietal pleurectomy is indicated. This can also be carried out endoscopically [13]. The first thoracoscopic reports on surgical treatment of pneumothorax were presented by Inderbitzi, who used endoligature [3]. Thoracotomy was a

**Table 1.** Patient characteristics and treatment

| Pat. no. Pneumothoraces | Age (years) | Sex | Localization (blebs) | Instrument | Follow-up | Histology (blebs) |
|---|---|---|---|---|---|---|
| 1 | 78 | M | Right lower lobe | E-scissor, fibrin | Subfebril (3rd–6th.d) 8 days | 2 ×1×1cm |
| 2 | 55 | F | Left upper lobe | 1× endo-GIA | 7 days | 3×2×2cm |
| 3 | 50 | F | Right upper lobe | 2× endo-GIA | 8 days | 3.5×1×1cm |
| 4 | 27 | M | Right upper lobe | 5× endo-GIA | 7 days | 5×4×2cm |
| 5 | 32 | M | Right upper lobe | 3× endo-GIA | 6 days | 5×4×3cm |
| 6 | 45 | M | Right upper lobe | 3× endo-GIA | 4 days | 3×3×2cm |
| 7 | 29 | M | – | 2× endo-GIA | 4 days | 5×3×2cm parenchyma, sarcoidosis |
| 8 | 46 | M | – | 2× endo-GIA | 4 days | 3×3×2cm parenchyma, silicosis |
| 9 | 71 | F | – | 3× endo-GIA | 4 days | 5×3×2cm sarcoidosis |
| 10 | 50 | M | – | 2× endo-GIA | 4 days | 4×1×1cm parenchyma sarcoidosis |
| 11 | 29 | M | – | 3× endo-GIA | 4 days | 4×3×2cm parenchyma, tuberculoma (15mm) |
| 12 | 78 | M | – | 8× endo-GIA | fever (3rd–7th d) 9 days | 8×8×4cm parenchyma, carcinoma (4.5cm) |
| 13 | 53 | M | – | 3× endo-GIA | 6 days | 4×3×3cm parenchyma, hamartoma (2,5cm) |
| 14 | 50 | M | – | 5× endo-GIA | 8 days | 7×4×2cm parenchyma tuberculoma (1,5cm) |
| 15 | 43 | M | – | E-scissor | 4 days | 5×5cm cyst wall ("unroofing") |

requirement of surgery until recently in the presence of large bullae (Elfeldt). It is thus to be assumed that the possibilities of minimally invasive techniques will also set new gold standards here [1].

**Systemic Diseases.** The diagnosis was confirmed by taking histological material (1× sarcoidosis, 3× silicosis). The technique specified by Greschuchna and Maassen [2,7, 8] with a 4-cm-long incision is of course almost as atraumatic and is to be considered invasive [11]. The possibility of exploring the entire pleural cavity is to be regarded as an advantage of the closed thoracoscopic procedure.

**Tumors.** The possibility of subsequent thoracotomy with traditional lung surgery when the result of the rapid section is positive is a precondition in the case of a tumor. In our patients, two tuberculomas, a hamartoma, and a cystic process were involved. The adenocarcinoma resected into healthy tissue in a 78-year-old colleague (patient number 12) did not entail any further consequences for us. It may be assumed that the development in the field of thoracoscopic surgery will continue until it involves lobectomy.

An important aspect of minimally invasive atypical peripheral lung resection (wedge resection) appears to us to be that thoracoscopic resection may constitute an alternative to conventional therapy – and one which facilitates the decision to operate in the case of unclear peripheral tumor. The latter is often the object of observation for many years, which entails considerable risk. We hope that surgeons will consider the possibility of endoscopic surgery, to which little attention has been paid up to now.

## *References*

1. Elfeldt R, Schroder D, Beske C (1989) Indikationen und Grenzen der Thorakoskopie bei der chirurgischen Diagnostik und Therapie von Lungenerkrankungen. Zentralbl. Chir. 114 (5): 281–285
2. Greschuchna D (1980) Indikationen der modifizierten chirurgischen Lungen- und Pleurabiopsie nach Maaben für die Differentialdiagnose disseminierter Lungenerkrankungen. Prax. Klin. Pneumol 34: 517
3. Inderbitzi R, Furrer M, Althaus V (1991) Die thorakoskopische Behandlung des Spontanpneumothorax. Ligatur durch chirurgischen Leckverschluß. Schweiz Med Wochenschr 121 [Suppl 36]: 18
4. Jacobäus HC (1910) Über die Möglichkeit die Zystoskopie bei Untersuchungen seröser Höhlen anzuwenden. Munch Med Wochenschr 57: 2090
5. Klassen KP, Anliyan AJ, Curtis GM (1949) Biopsy of diffuse pulmonary lesions. Arch. Surg. 59: 694
6. Kux E (1974) Thorakoskopische Eingriffe am Nervensystem. Thieme, Stuttgart
7. Maassen W (1989) Thorakoskopie: chirurgische Technik. Pneumologie 43: 53–54
8. Maassen W (1972) Direkte Thorakoskopie ohne vorherige oder mögliche Pneumothoraxanlage. Endoscopy 4: 95
9. Sattler A (1969) Warum ist die Thorakoskopie zur Durchführung einer kausalen Therapie schwerer Fälle von Spontanpneumothorax indiziert? Presented at the 11th Wissenschaftlichen Tagung der Norddeutschen Gesellschaft für Tuberkulose und Lungenkrankheit, 19 Oct 1969
10. Sattler A (1944) Zur Endoskopie der tuberkulösen Kaverne am Lebenden. Wien Klin Wochenschr 59: 41
11. Schaberg T, Suttmann-Bayerl A, Loddenkemper R (1989) Thorakoskopie bei diffusen Lungenkrankheiten. Pneumologie 43 (2): 112–115
12. Takeno Y (1987) Thoracoscopic therapy for the patients with spontaneous pneumothorax. Respir Res (Tokyo) 6: 823–829
13. Wieser O, Wieser CO (1989) Indikationen zur Thorakoskopie beim sekundären Spontanpneumothorax. Pneumologie 43 (2): 92–95
14. Wittmoser R (1961) Thoraxchirurgie: Fehler und Gefahren der thorakoskopischen Denervation. Chir Praxis 1: 79–92

# Liver Biopsy: Modified Menghini and Trucut Needles for Fibrin Sealing of the Biopsy Channel: Clinical Experience

G. JUDMAIER, W. VOGEL, H. P. DINGES, and K. ZATLOUKAL

## Abstract

Histologic investigation of liver tissue obtained by percutaneous needle biopsy remains the mainstay in the diagnosis of liver disease. Impaired blood clotting or thrombocytopenia precludes percutaneous liver biopsy for the danger of sometimes life-threatening hemorrhage as the most serious complication. The feasibility of plugging the intrahepatic needle track with fibrin sealant to minimize the risk of bleeding has been shown. The advantage of the method presented here is that biopsy and sealing can be performed as a one-step procedure, thus shortening the time necessary and minimizing the risk of complications. We considered laparoscopic control most reliable to optimize handling of the double-channel needles and to assess the reliability of fibrin plugging for the "blind" percutaneous approach. In 27 patients a modified Menghini needle and in 10 patients a modified Trucut needle were tested. In our experience the handling of the modified Trucut needle proved easier. There was, however, no significant difference in the length of the biopsy core obtained with the two needles (16 ± 8.6 mm Menghini needle and 15.75 ± 7.1 mm Trucut needle), resulting from the larger diameter of the Menghini needle (1.8). The thin trickle of bleeding observed around the plug in a few patients was without clinical significance, reflecting the prolonged coagulation time in these patients. In summary, in the hands of an experienced investigator the combined biopsy-plugging device is a safe and reliable tool for obtaining liver tissue in patients with impaired blood coagulation. As a one-step procedure it can be performed quickly, thus increasing safety by diminishing the need for patient cooperation.

## Introduction

Histologic investigation of liver tissue remains the mainstay in the diagnosis of liver disease. Impaired blood clotting or thrombocytopenia precludes percutaneous liver biopsy for the danger of sometimes life-threatening hemorrhage as the most serious complication [1]. The feasibility of plugging the intrahepatic needle track with fibrin sealant to minimize the risk of bleeding has been shown [2]. Previously, it has been demonstrated [3–5] that plugging the needle track with gelfoam or fibrin in patients with impaired clotting is safe. These reported methods, however, have the disadvantage of leaving a cannula within the liver tissue for the application of fibrin after removing obturator and specimen. Therefore, a device was developed [6] allowing the biopsy to be performed as a one-step procedure with application of a fibrin sealant (Tissucol) while withdrawing the needle from the liver. We considered laparascopic control most reliable to optimize handling of the double-channel needles and to assess the reliability of fibrin plugging for the "blind" percutaneous approach.

## Patients and Methods

In 27 patients the modified Menghini needle and in 10 patients the modified Trucut needle were tested. All patients underwent peritoneoscopic investigations for reasons unrelated to the present study. Abnormal clotting time and a low thrombocyte count precluding percutaneous biopsy were the reasons for the laparoscopic biopsy approach in 22 cirrhotic patients. The other 15 patients underwent laparoscopic investigation for staging of malignant disease. Liver biopsy was performed via a second percutaneous approach, and the needle movements were guided under direct laparoscopic control. The only difference to a conventional biopsy procedure was that the needle had to be removed from the liver more slowly while injecting the activated fibrin sealant through the attached Duploject syringe. The fibrin sealant was applied through the small outer channel of the double-channeled needle. The modified Menghini needle had an external diameter of 2.1 mm and the biopsy channel 1.8 mm, the Trucut needle 2.5 mm and 2.1 mm, respectively.

## Results

Handling of the Menghini needle proved technically more demanding and the specimens were lost in five patients because the tissue core sealed into the biopsy channel. No problems were encountered with the Trucut needle. In two cases the Menghini technique failed to provide tissue at the first biopsy attempt. Liver tissue obtained with both needles yielded good material for histologic investigation, with a variation in sample length of $15 \pm 8.65$ mm. Bleeding had to be stopped once by electrocoagulation after plugging had failed due to a defective prototype Menghini needle. Minimal local bleeding was observed around the successfully applied fibrin plug in three patients of the Menghini group without correlation to underlying disease or clotting results. All Trucut biopsies were successful, with effective plugging of the biopsy channel. None of the patients had any problems in holding the breath for rapid biopsy performance. No additional pain during the biopsy procedure or after closing the abdomen was reported. Hemoglobin levels were stable over a 6-h observation period.

## Discussion

Laparoscopic or transvenous liver biopsies are so far the only feasible methods for obtaining liver tissue in patients at a high risk of bleeding. However, these investigations are available only in specialized centers and have the drawback of providing only small specimens [7]. The feasibility of plugging the intrahepatic needle track with fibrin sealant has been shown previously [3–5] by means of a second access by leaving either a sheath or cannula in situ. The advantage of the method presented here is that biopsy and sealing can be performed as a one-step procedure, thus shortening the necessary time and minimizing the risk of complications. We considered laparoscopic control most reliable for optimizing the handling of the double-channel needles for assessing the reliability of fibrin plugging for the "blind" percutaneous approach, and for testing the biopsy system in patients with high risk of bleeding. In our hands the handling of the modified Trucut needle proved easier, and the tissue produced was sufficient for morphological investigation. There was, however, no significant difference in the length of the biopsy core obtained with the two needles. The only plugging failure occurred with a defective prototype Menghini needle. In a few patients a thin trickle of bleeding was observed around the plug but without clinical significance. In summary, in the hands of an experienced investigator the combined biopsy-plugging device is a safe and reliable tool for obtaining liver tissue in patients with impaired blood coagulation, and the first experiences employing this device without laparoscopic control in patients with abnormal clotting tests confirm the reported results. As a one-step procedure it can be performed quickly, thus increasing safety by diminishing the need for patient cooperation.

## References

1. Lindner H (1967) Grenzen und Gefahren der perkutanen Leberbiopsie mit der Menghininadel. Dtsch med Wochenschr 92: 1751–1757
2. Hegarty JE, Williams R (1984) Liver biopsy: techniques, clinical application and complication. Br Med J 288: 1254–1256
3. Riley SA, Ellis WR, Irving HC, Lintott DJ, Axon ATR, Losowsky MS (1984) Percutaneous liver biopsy with plugging of needle track: a safe method for use in patients with impaired coagulation. Lancet ii: 436
4. Chisholm RA, Jones SN, Lees WR (1989) Fibrin sealant as a plug for the post liver biopsy needle track. Clin Radiol 40: 627–628
5. Tobin MV, Gilmore IT (1989) Plugged liver biopsy in patients with impaired coagulation. Dig Dis Sci 34: 13–15
6. Zatloukal K, Dinges HP, Thurnher M, Redl H, Schlag G (1988) A new technique of liver biopsy with plugging of the needle track using a double channel biopsy device. Z Gastroenterol 26: 699–703
7. Lebrec D, Goldfarb G, Degott C, Rueff B, Benhamou J (1982) Transvenous liver biopsy. Gastroenterology 83: 338–340

# Subject Index

abdominoperineal rectum extirpation 38
abortions, intrauterine 87
abscess
– perianastomotic 33
– perirectal 79
acid output
– basal (BAO) 22
– peak (PAO) 22
adrenalin 13
– adrenalin / polidocanol, combination 15
air embolism, risk of 42
alimentary tract, fistulae 50, 55
– lower tract 55
amelioration by the sealing therapy 76
ampullary anastomoses 84
anal fistulas in Crohn's disease (see also
  Crohn's disease) 75 ff.
– age ranges 76
– defunctioning colostomy 76
– perianal fistulas 75
– surgical treatment 75
anastomoses / anastomotic defects
– ampullary 84
– anastomotic stenosis 34
– endoscopic application of fibrin
  glue 33 ff.
– endogastrointestinal anastomosis 101
– esophagojejunal anastomoses 53
– isthmic 84
– laparoscopic colon anastomosis 40, 42
– lower gastrointestinal tract 34
– postoperative 35
– reliable anastomotic technique 38
– Roux-en-Y-anastomosis 34
– tubal 84
– upper gastrointestinal tract 33
angiogenetic effect of fibrin sealant, solitary rectal ulcer syndrome 73
anti-inflammatory drugs 76
antibiogram, fistula secretion 59
antibiotics 26, 51, 55, 59, 76, 79

– septic complications with antibiotic prophylaxis, postoperative fistulas 79, 80
antiseptic surgery 35
antropyloric
– motility 21
– pump 21
appendicitis 24
application, fibrin glue
– injection therapy (see also there) 1 ff.,
  8 ff., 11 ff., 44, 51, 59, 69 ff.
– intravasal 45
– paravasal 45
– spray application 42
– submucosal 15 ff.
aprotinin 71
ASA III patient 20
aspiration 22, 55
– into the bronchial system 52
azathioprim 65


babies, gastrointestinal fistulas 50, 52
bacteria / bacterial contamination, colonic 40, 42
betnesol 76
bile ducts, fibrin sealing 32
biliary
– cyst 24
– drainage 79
– fistulas 58, 78–80
– secretions 79
biliary-cutaneous fistulas 79
biopsy, liver (see also liver) 106–108
bleeding
– after rectum excision 40
– esophageal varices (see also there) 44,
  45
– – acute 45
– – re-bleeding 44
– gastroduodenal ulcer hemorrhage 1–3,
  8, 9
– – arterial bleeders 5

– – non-variceal 2
– – oozing bleeding (Forrest Ib) 8, 9
– – re-bleeding (*see also there*) 4, 9
– – relapses 15
– – sphincterotomy 15
– – spurting bleeding (Forrest Ia) 8, 9
– – visible vessel (Forrest IIa) 8, 9
– gallbladder fossa 31
– gynecological surgery, endoscopic 92
– liver biopsy 107
blood
– coagulation disorder 9
– staunching, mechanical (Senkstaken-
  Blakermore tube) 44
– tests, before and after sclerotherapy 47
– transfusion
– – gastroduodenal ulcer hemorrhage 8,
  11
– – sclerotherapy, esophageal varices 47
bowel
– fistula, endoscopic gynecological
  surgery 82
– infectious 75
– inflammatory diseases 76, 79
bronchial
– fistulas 60, 75
– system, aspiration 52
bronchoesophageal fistulas 55
bronchoscope 52


cannula
– double lumen 10
– positions 10
– single-lumen 10
carcinoma
– lung (*see there*)
– gastric (*see also there*) 1, 2, 15–17
– rectum, lower rectum 40
cardiac ulcers 2
cavum retzii
– endoscopic preparation 96
– visualization 97
chemical lesions 16
children endoscopic therapy 50
cholecystectomy 23, 25, 103
– laparoscopic (LCHE; *see also*
  liver bed) 30 ff.
cholecystitis 24
closure of perforated ulcer 25, 26
clotting
– luminal 46
– proteins, plasmatic 71
$CO_2$
– embolism 27
– insufflation 97
– pneumocavus 98

coagulation 8, 12
– blood coagulation disorders 9, 31
– electrocoagulation / electrocautery (*see
  also there*) 8, 12, 13, 16, 23, 51
– laser coagulation (*see also* laser) 8, 12,
  16, 23, 24, 44
colifoam 76
colonic
– bacteria 40
– interposition after esophageal
  resection 33
– lavage 40, 55
– wall lesions 50
colorectal
– fistulas 33, 35
– operations / surgery (*see also* laparoscopic colorectal surgery) 33, 34, 38 ff.
colostomy 39, 40
– defunctioning 76
– traction-free establishment 39
corticosteroids 76
costs 78
– sclerotherapy (*see also there*) 48
Crohn's disease (*see also* fistulas) 55, 56,
  58, 62, 63, 65 ff.
– anal fistulas (*see also there*) 75 ff.
– complication of the underlying disease 65 ff.
– conservative therapy 65
– formula diets 65
– inflammation activity 66
– occlusion of fistulas (*see also there*) 58 ff, 65 ff.
– parenteral nutrition 65
– patients psychological state 66
– perianal fistulas 75
– surgical therapy 65
cyanoacrylate 51, 52
cyclosporin 65
cystojejunostomy 79
cytology brush 51


death causes
– gastroduodenal ulcer hemorrhage 11,
  27
– liver diseases 44
– occlusion of fistulas 62
débridement, endoscopically, fistulas 60
diarrhea 27, 66
– postoperative 21
diet (*see also* nutrition)
– formular 65
– high-fiber-diet 70
– hygienic-dietary measures 70, 71
Dieulafoy ulcer 2
Doppler sonography 9

drainage fluids, postoperative  32
duodenal
– ulcer (*see* gastroduodenal ulcer)
– wall lesions  20

echinococcosis, hepatic  79
electro-hydro-thermal probe  8
electrocoagulation (APE) / electrocautery  8, 12, 13, 16, 23, 51
– bipolar  12
– wound margins  51
embolism risk
– air  42
– CO2  27
– gas  42
– pulmonary  47
embolization, endoscopic  17
emergency
– endoscopy for bleeding  4, 9–12
– surgery, gastroduodenal ulcer hemorrhage  8, 10
endocrine tumors  79
endogastrointestinal anastomosis, minimally invasive lung surgery  101
endometriosis  69, 73, 90
– pelvic  72
endoprosthesis implantation, gastrointestinal fistulas  53
endoscopic
– cautering  34
– **fibrin sealing**
– – advantages  35
– – anal fistulas (*see also there*)  75 ff.
– – anastomotic defects  33 ff.
– – esophageal varices, sclerotherapy
  (*see also* sclerotherapy)  44 ff.
– – fistulas  33 ff.
– – gastroduodenal ulcer hemorrhage
  (*see also there*)  1 ff., 8 ff.
– – gynecological surgery (*see also* there)  82 ff., 90 ff.
– – injection therapy (*see there*)
– – laparoscopic surgical treatment
  (*see also there*)  20 ff., 38 ff.
– – liver bed after laparoscopic cholecystectomy (*see also there*)  30 ff.
– – liver biopsy (*see also there*)  106 ff.
– – lung surgery (*see also there*)  100 ff.
– – Marshall-Marchetti-Krantz-Operation
  (MMKH; *see also there*)  96 ff.
– – minimally invasive surgery
  (*see also there*)  100 ff.
– – perforation  33 ff.
– – occlusion of fistulas
  (*see also there*)  58 ff.

– – solitary rectal ulcer syndrome
  (*see also there*)  69 ff.
– – submucosal fibrin adhesion (*see also*
  *there*)  15 ff.
– hemostasis  8, 15, 17
endoscopy
– emergency  4, 9–12
– re-endoscopy  10, 16
epinephrine  2, 4, 8
– fibrin sealant (FS) / hypertonic saline
  with epinephrine (HSE), combination
  (HSE/FS)  2
– local injection  8
– polidocanol / epinephrine,
  combination  4, 9, 12
– preliminary injection  8
erythrocyte concentrates  11
esophageal
– anastomotic leakage  50
– atresia  50, 52
– fistulas  75
– mucosal damage  45
– perforations  53
– resection and reconstruction  33, 36
– – colonic interposition after  33
– ulcer hemorrhage  15–17
– – caused by sclerotherapy  44, 47
– varices / variceal  9, 44 ff., 71
– – bleeding (*see also there*)  45
– – sclerosis  71
– – sclerotherapy (*see also*
  sclerotherapy)  44 ff.
esophagitis  15, 16
esophagogastric leakages  53
esophagogastro-duodenoscopy  2
esophagogastrostomy  33
esophagojejunal anastomoses  53
esophagojejunostomy  79
esophagotracheal fistulas, congenital  52
ethanolaminoleate  45

feeding (*see also* nutrition)  41
fertilization, laparoscopic refertilization  91, 93
**fibrin**
– clot, submucosal  4
– collagen application  25
– fibrin glue / fibrin sealing, endoscopic
  (*see also* endoscopic fibrin sealing)
– FS / HSE, combination (HSE/FS)  2
fibrinogen / thrombin, combination  58
fibrinolytic drugs  59
fibroblasts, ingrowth  51
Fisher's exact test  10
fistula secretion  63
– antibiogram  59

fistulas
- alimentary tract  50, 55
- biliary (*see also there*)  58, 78–80
- bronchial  60
- bronchoesophageal  55
- chronic  34
- classification  62, 63
- colorectal  33, 35
- Crohn's disease (*see also there*)  62, 63
- endoscopic application of fibrin
  glue  33 ff., 50
- enteroenteral and enterocutaneous  55,
  67
- enterovesical  67
- esophageal  75
- esophagotracheal, congenital  52
- gallbladder  59
- gastrocutaneous fistula  79
- gastrointestinal (*see also there*)  50 ff.,
  58–60, 78, 80
- occlusion, endoscopic approaches
  (*see also* occlusion)  58 ff., 65
- occurence of  66
- pancreatic  78–80
- postoperative (*see also there*)  78 ff.
- pulmonary  60
- radiogenic  54
- rectovaginal  33–35, 62, 65–67
- respiratory tract  50, 58
- septic  59
- small intestine  59
- stomalike  59
- tracheobronchial  50, 60
- tumor  59
- vaginal (*see also there*)  78–80
- vaginosacral  62
fistuloscopy  58–63
fluoroscopic control, postoperative
  fistulas  80
Forrest (F) classifications, gastroduodenal ulcer hemorrhage  1, 2, 8, 9
- F Ia (spurting bleeding)  8, 9
- F Ia/b  2
- F Ib (oozing bleeding)  8, 9
- F Iia (visible vessel)  8, 9
- F IIa/b  2
- F III  1
fresh human plasma  45


gallbladder
- bleeding from the gallbladder fossa  31
- fistulas  59
- hemostasis  30
- laparoscopic dissection (*see also* liver
  bed)  30, 31
gallstones  30

gas embolism, risk of  42
gastrectomy  33, 79
gastric
- carcinoma / cancer  1, 2, 15–17, 79
- - arterial bleeding  17
- - benign ulcers  1, 2
- nerves  20
gastroduodenal ulcer hemorrhage  1 ff.,
  8 ff., 20 ff.
- application (*see also* injection therapy)
- bleeding (*see also there*)  1–3, 8, 9
- chronic  26
- death causes  11
- duodenal wall lesions  20
- emergency
- - endoscopy for bleeding  4, 9–12
- - surgery  8, 10
- endoscopic injection therapy  1, 2, 4, 8,
  11, 12
- Forrest classification (*see also there*)
  1, 2
- laparoscopic surgical treatment (*see
  also there*)  20 ff.
- morbidity  27
- mortality rate  1, 4, 8, 12, 15
- motility (*see also there*)  21
- multiorgan failure  3
- necroses  3
- perforated ulcer  22, 26, 27
- - closure of perforated ulcer  25, 26
- perforation risk  10
- randomized comparison of fibrin sealant vs. polidocanol  8 ff.
- re-bleeding (*see also there*)  4, 9
- re-endoscopy  10, 16
- sclerotherapy (*see also there*)  4, 8, 9,
  12, 16
- surgical interventions  3
- upper gastrointestinal
- - hemorrhage (*see also there*)  3, 15
- - tract (*see also there*)  33
- variceal bleeding  2
gastroesophageal reflux  27
gastrografin passage  34
gastrointestinal fistulas, fibrin sealant
  therapy  50 ff., 58–60, 78, 80
- babies  50, 52
- congenital fistulas  52
- cutaneous fistula  79
- endoprosthesis implantation  53
- endoscopic fistula treatment  50
- esophagogastric leakages  53
- esophagojejunal anastomoses  53
- indications for endoscopic sealing  51,
  52, 55
- infection, chronic  51, 56
- inflammatory fistula, chronic  56

– injection therapy  51
– lower gastrointestinal tract  59
– postoperative fistulas  53
– properties  51
– radiogenic defects  54, 56
– radiotherapy  51
– results  52
– traumatic esophageal fistulas  53
– tumor fistulae  50, 51, 55, 56
– upper gastrointestinal tract  59
glue mixture
– glue of thrombin and fibrinogen  58
– just before application  33
granulation tissue  35
gynecological surgery, endoscopic, fibrin
  sealant  82 ff., 90 ff.
– bleedings  82
– bowel fistula  82
– conditions  91
– endoscopic myomectomy (*see also*
  *there*)  82, 83
– fibrin sealing
– – advantages  94
– – disadvantages  94
– hemostasis in surgical intervention  90 ff.
– instruments  82
– laparoscopic refertilization  91
– neovagina, endoscopically assisted
  (*see also there*)  88, 99
– Mayer-Rokitansky-Küster (MRK)
  syndrome  88
– myoma enucleation  94
– salpingotomy  91
– second-look laparoscopies  94
– tubal anastomosis (*see also the-*
  *re*)  84–88, 90
– ulcera  82

hamartoma, lung  105
Hartmann's operation  79
heart failure  11
heater probe  16
hematemesis  9
hemofiltration  34
hemorrhagic complications, postoperative
  fistulas  79
hemostasis  1, 30, 41
– endoscopic  8, 15, 17
– gallbladder  30, 32
– laparoscopic colorectal surgery  41, 42
– permanent  5
– in surgical intervention  90 ff.
hepatectomy  79
hepatic
– echinococcosis  79

– metastases  40
hepatitis
– B virus  45
– C virus  45
hiatal area, laparoscopic treatment  24
histoacryl  17, 45, 50
HSE (hypertonic saline with
  epinephrine)  4
– fibrin sealant (FS) / hypertonic saline
  with epinephrine(HSE)  2
hygienic-dietary measures  70, 71
hypertension
– intraabdominal  93
– portal  31
hypotension  9
hysterectomy, vaginal fistula after  79
hysteroscopy  87

ileostomy  76
– Kock's reservoir  79, 80
imflammatory bowel disease  76
incisura
– angularis  21
– cardiaca  21
infections
– chronic  35, 51
– – gastrointestinal fistulas  51, 56
– colonic bacteria  40, 42
– infectious bowel  75
inflammation activity, Crohn's disease
  66
inflammatory bowel disease  79
injection therapy of fibrin glue
– endoscopic  1–4, 8, 11–13, 70, 71
– – sclerotomy (*see also there*)  44
– gastrointestinal fistulas  51
– intramural  59
– intravariceal  16
– intravascular  16
– submucosal  16
– transendoscopic  16
insulinoma  79
intraabdominal hypertension  93
intramural injection of fibrin glue  59
intrathoracic complications after esophageal and stomach surgery  33
isthmic anastomoses  84
isthmoampullary tubal pregnancy  91–93

Kock's reservoir ileostomy  79, 80
laparatomy, re-laparatomy  35
laparoscopic
– colorectal surgery  38 ff.
– – anastomosis of colon, laparoscopic  40, 42

– – animal study 40
– – clinical study 40
– – complications 38, 40
– – embolism 42
– – diffuse bleeding 40
– – indications for fibrin sealing 40
– – minimally invasive procedure 38
– – oncological radicality, principles 38
– – rectum extirpation / excision (*see also*
    *there*) 38–40
– – retropexy technique (*see also*
    *there*) 38, 39, 42
– – time of operation, reduces 42
– – tissue rupture 42
– linear salpingotomy in isthmoampullary
    tubal pregnancy 91–93
– refertilization 91, 93
– surgical treatment, duodenal ulcer dis-
    ease 20 ff.
– – hiatal area 24
– – indications 22
– – instrumentation 23
– – liver bed after laparoscopic cholecys-
    tectomy (*see also there*) 30 ff.
– – patient position 23
– – patient selection 22
– – principles of the operation 20
– vagotomy, laparoscopic 22
– video-laparoscopic intervention 22
laser coagulation 8, 12, 16, 23, 24, 44
– Nd-YAG-laser systems 23, 24
Latarjet's nerve 21
liver
– bed after laparoscopic
    chloecystectomy 30 ff.
– – drainage fluids, postoperative 32
– – sealing of the liver bed 32
– – ultrasononographic evaluation 31
– biopsy 106–108
– – bleeding 107
– – histologic investigation 107
– – laparoscopic 108
– – Menghini needle 106–108
– – percutaneous needle biopsy 106
– – thrombocytopenia 106
– – transvenous 108
– – Trucut needle 108
– diseases 44, 45
– – child's classification 45
– – death after liver failure 44
– – liver cirrhosis 44
lobectomy 102
lower gastrointestinal tract, anastomotic
    defects 34
lung
– carcinoma 102
– – adenocarcinoma 102, 105

– cystic process 105
– hamartoma 105
– minimally invasive surgery 100 ff.
– – endogastrointestinal anastomosis 101
– – pneumothorax, spontaneous 100
– – pulmonary resection 100, 105
– – technique 100–102
– resection (wedge resection) 105
– surgery, thoracoscopic 103
lymph node dissection 38


malignoma 11
Mallory-Weiss tear 15, 16
Marshall-Marchetti-Krantz-Operation
    (MMKH) 96 ff.
– cavum retzii (*see also there*) 96, 97
– minimally invasive surgery 98
– retrosymphysial area 97
– urinary stress incontinence 96
Mayer-Rokitansky-Küster (MRK) syn-
    drome 88
Menghini needle, liver biopsy 106–108
6-mercaptopurine 65
mesocolon, mobilization 39
metastases
– hepatic 40
– pulmonary 40
methylene blue 71
metromidazole 65
midazolam 46
minimally invasive surgery 98, 100 ff.
– endoscopic MMKH 98
– laparoscopic colorectal surgery 38, 39
– lung surgery (*see also there*) 100 ff.
morbidity
– gastroduodenal ulcer hemorrhage 27
– liver cirrhosis 44
mortality rate
– gastroduodenal ulcer hemorrhage 1, 4,
    8, 12, 15
– liver cirrhosis 44, 45
– postoperative fistulas 78
motility, antropyloric 21
mucorrhage 70, 72
multiorgan failure 3
myoma enucleation 94
myomectomy, endoscopic 82, 83
– principles 83
– results by laparatomy and laparosco-
    py 83


Nd-YAG laser coagulation 24
necrosis
– gastroduodenal ulcer hemorrhage 3
– pancreatitis, necrotizing 79

– occlusion of fistulas  62, 63
necrotic cavities, fistulas  60
neovagina, endoscopically assisted  88, 89
– operative technique  88
– results  88
nerves
– gastric  20
– Latarjet's  21
– secretory  20
– vagus (see also there)  21
nutrition  41, 52, 55, 65, 78, 80
– formular diets  65
– nutrition tube  52, 53
– parenteral  55, 65, 78, 80

occlusion of fistulas, endoscopic approaches  58 ff.
– anal fistulas (see also there)  75 ff.
– Crohn's disease (see also there)  58, 65
– duration and outcome of treatment  61
– follow-up examination  62
– iatrogenic injuries  61
– necroses  61
– number of gluings and result  61
– wound healing disorder  58
occurrence of fistulas  66
omental flap  20
omeprazole  4, 16
oncological radicality, principles, laparoscopic colorectal surgery  38
osteomyelites  96
ovaries, reshaping  91
ovarian cyst extirpation  91

pain, postoperative  23, 25
pancreatic
– cancer  79, 80
– fistulas  78–80
– pseudocyst marsupialization  79
– secretions  79
pancreaticoduodenectomy  80
pancreatitis, necrotizing  79
parasympathetic territory, posterior  21
pelvic endometriosis  72, 73
pentazocine  46
peptic ulcer hemorrhage (see also gastroduodenal ulcer)  1 ff., 8 ff., 15 ff.
perforated ulcer  22, 27
– endoscopic application of fibrin glue  33 ff.
– iatrogenic  34
– perforation risk  10
periostites  96
peritoneal damage  93

– hemostatic purposes  93
– reparation  93
– uterovesical  88
peritonitis  22, 34
– chemical  22
Pfannenstiels incision  96
plasma clotting proteins  71
pneumoperitoneum  23
pneumothorax  27, 100–103
polidocanol  16, 46
– adrenalin / polidocanol, combination  15
– fibrin sealant vs. polidocanol, randomized comparison of  8 ff.
– injection  12, 13
– – intravariceal injection  44
– polidocanol / epinephrine, combination  4, 9, 12
– occlusion of fistulas  59
polypectomy  71
polypoid lesions, rectal ulcer syndrome  70–72
portocaval shunt operation  45
postoperative fistulas, human fibrin sealants  78 ff.
– conservative therapy  79
– costs  78
– delayed  78
– drainage position  79
– early  78
– fluoroscopic control  80
– hemorrhagic complications  79
– mortality rate  78
– parenteral nutrition  78
– septic complications with antibiotic prophylaxis  79, 80
pregnancy  9
– intrauterine  87
proctalgia  70
prolamine sulfate  51
prolapse of the rectum  38, 41, 69, 70
– prolapse correction  70
psychological state, Crohn's disease  66
pulmonary
– embolism  47
– fistulas  60
– metastases  40
– resection  100
pyloric spasm  21

radiogenic fistulas  54
radiopaque, hydrosoluble  80
radiotherapy, gastrointestinal fistulas  51, 56
randomized comparison of fibrin sealant vs. polidocanol  8 ff.

ranitidine 16
rats 16
re-bleeding
– esophageal varices, sclerotherapy 44
– gastroduodenal, ulcer hemorrhage 4, 9
– – clinical signs 9
– – rate of 4
re-endoscopy 10, 16
re-laparatomy 35
re-thoracotomy 35
rectal
– carcinoma 38
– fibrosis 73
rectorrhage 70, 72
rectovaginal fistulas 33–35, 65, 66
– conservative therapy 66
– effectiveness of fistula therapy 67
rectum
– abscess, perirectal 79
– carcinoma, lower rectum 40
– extirpation / excision, laparoscopic
    abdominoperineal 38–40
– – abdominal excision 40
– – anterior dissection 39
– – diffuse bleeding after 40
– – operative procedure 39
– – palliative excision 40
– – time of operation, reduces 42
– – vaginosacral fistula 62
– mobilization 39
– prolapse (see also there) 38, 41, 69,
    70
– solitary rectal ulcer syndrome (see also
    there) 69 ff.
respiratory
– failure 27
– fistulae 50, 58
retropexy technique, laparoscopic colo-
    rectal surgery 38 ff.
– experimental study 42
– with marlex mesh 42
– operative procedure 39
– Well's rectopexy 38, 39, 41
retrosymphysial area 97
retziusscopy 96–98
Roux-en-Y-anastomosis 34


saline, hypertrophic with epinephrine
    (HSE) / fibrin sealant (FS), combina-
    tion (HSE/FS) 2
salpingotomy 91
– in isthmoampullary tubal pregnancy,
    laparoscopic 91–93
sclerotherapy
– esophageal varices (see also
    there) 44 ff.

– – blood tests before and after sclerothe-
    rapy 47
– – contraindication for shunt therapy 48
– – costs 48
– – erosions 48
– – esophageal ulcers caused by sclero-
    therapy 44
– – fever complications 44
– – injection sclerotherapy 45
– – intravariceal fibrin injection 44
– – local complications 48
– – prophylactic 48
– – thromboembolic complications 44
– – treatment scheme 46
– – ulcerations 48
– gastroduodenal ulcer hemorrhage (see
    also there) 4, 8, 9, 12, 16
second-look surgery, postoperative fistu-
    las 78
secretions, aggressive 79
– biliary 79
– pancreatic 79
secretive tests 22
secretory nerves 20
Senkstaken-Blakermore tube, mechanical
    blood staunching 44, 45, 47
septic
– complications 34
– – with antibiotic prophylaxis, postoper-
    ative fistlulas 79
– fistulas 59
seromuscular layer 21
seromyotomy, anterior 20–22, 24, 25, 27, 28
shunt operation 44, 45
– contraindication for sclerotherapy 48
– portocaval shunt 45
sigmoid colon 39
small intestine fistulas 59
solitary rectal ulcer syndrome 69 ff.
– angiogenetic effect of fibrin sealant 73
– large elevated ulcers 69, 72
– – at times with polypoid formations 72
– polypoid lesions 70, 71
– small and superficial ulcers 69, 71, 72
– Tissucol injection 69
– treatment 69, 72
somatostatin 59, 78
– fistulas 59
sphincterotomy bleeding 15, 16
stomalike fistulas 59
stool
– bloody 9
– tarry 9
Student's t-test 31
submucosal fibrin adhesion 15 ff.
– complications 15
surgery, open 20, 24

tachycardia  9
Tayler's procedure  20–22, 25, 28
tenesmus  70
thermal energy, application of  8, 9
thermic
– lesions  16
– procedures  44
thoracal / thoracic
– intrathoracic complications after esophageal and stomach surgery  33
– re-thoracotomy  35
thoracocentesis  100
thoracoscopy / thoracotomy, lung surgery
  (*see also* lung)  100–105
thorax
– constricted  102
– drain  102
thrombin / fibrinogen, combination  58
thrombocytopenia  106
Tissucol (two-component system)  50
– endoscopic gynecological surgery  82
– solitary rectal ulcer syndrome (*see also*
  *there*)  69 ff.
tissue damage  15
tracheal fistulas  60
tracheobronchial fistulae  50
transendoscopic injection therapy  16
transfusion, gastroduodenal ulcer hemorrhage  8, 11
Trasylol (two-component system)  51
triflupromazine  46
trocars insertion for video-
  laparoscope  23
Trucut needle, liver biopsy  108
tubal
– anastomosis  84–88, 90
– – operative technique  84
– – principles  85
– – results  84, 85
– pregnancy, isthmoampullary  91–93
tuberculomas  105
tuberculosis  69, 72, 73
tumors
– endocrine  79
– tumor fistulae, gastrointestinal  50, 55,
  56
– – sealing of  51


ulcers
– duodeni / duodenal (*see also* gastroduodenal ulcer)  1 ff., 8 ff.
– esophageal  15

– vaginitis, ulcerous  66
– ventriculi  10
ultrasonographic evaluation, liver bed  31
upper gastrointestinal
– hemorrhage  3, 15
– tract, anastomotic defect  33
urinary stress incontinence, Marshall-
  Marchetti-Krantz-Operation
  (MMKH)  96 ff.
uterovesical peritoneum  88


vagina / vaginal
– fistulas  78–80
– neovagina, endoscopically assisted  88,
  89
vaginitis, ulcerous  66
vaginosacral fistula after rectal
  extirpation  62
vagotomy  21, 24, 26
– anterior  24
– laparoscopic  22
– selective  21
– posterior  24
– truncal, posterior  20–22, 24, 28
vagus nerves  21
– secretory branches  21
varices / variceal
– bleeding  2, 17
– esophageal (*see also there*)  9, 44 ff.
– intravariceal fibrin injection  16
– obliteration  47
varicose veins  45
vasoconstructiva  16
ventilation, mechanical  34, 52
video-laparoscopic intervention  22
– trocars insertion for  23


wedge resection, lung  105
Well's rectopexy  38, 39, 41
– transabdominal  39
wound healing  16, 27
– substrate phase  16


xiphoid probe  24


YAG laser systems  23

# Springer-Verlag
# and the Environment

We at Springer-Verlag firmly believe that an international science publisher has a special obligation to the environment, and our corporate policies consistently reflect this conviction.

We also expect our business partners – paper mills, printers, packaging manufacturers, etc. – to commit themselves to using environmentally friendly materials and production processes.

The paper in this book is made from low- or no-chlorine pulp and is acid free, in conformance with international standards for paper permanency.